HOW TO
Lower
Cholesterol
WITH ESSENTIAL OIL

HOW TO
Lower
Cholesterol
WITH ESSENTIAL OIL

By Rebecca Park Totilo

How to Lower Cholesterol With Essential Oil

Paperback ISBN: 978-0-9991865-1-0

Electronic ISBN: 978-0-9991865-2-7

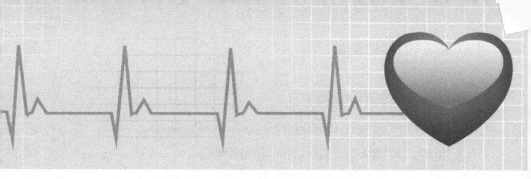

Contents

INTRODUCTION

Cholesterol is a natural function of the human body. In fact, all vertebrates need this waxy, fat-like substance that is found in all living cells in the body. It circulates throughout the blood to settle in body tissues and blood plasma in the form of fatty lipids (steroids) and alcohol. Cholesterol, therefore, is necessary to maintain and balance levels of hormones, vitamin D, and other substances to digest your food and the body has no problem making what it needs. However, the food we eat also contains cholesterol. The problem now is what happens to this additional or excess cholesterol that the body doesn't need?

Two kinds of lipoproteins carry cholesterol throughout the body: low-density lipoproteins (LDL) and high-density lipoproteins. The low-density lipoproteins or LDL is referred to as "bad cholesterol" that causes lipoproteins to act as the carrier molecules, and deposit LDL cholesterol on the walls of the arteries. It then thickens and hinders normal blood passage causing atherosclerosis. High-density lipoprotein, on the other hand, is considered "good cholesterol" because the HDL carries cholesterol from other parts of your body back to the liver where it is removed from your body. HDL cholesterol acts as an antioxidant, and helps to manufacture bile that aids to digest fats essential to the functions of fat-soluble vitamins A, D, E, and K. All these mentioned vitamins assist in the metabolism roles in the reproductive organs, from puberty developmental process until maturity, which also affects the estrogen level in the body.

PRIMARY SOURCES OF GOOD CHOLESTEROL

1. Three-fourth (75%) of good cholesterol comes from within the body or is produced internally through results from synthesizing densely packed membranes like liver, central nervous system (spinal cord, includes brain), reproductive organs, adrenal gland, and atheroma. The degenerative changes in the atheroma result to the development of atherosclerotic plaques and coronary artery disease that affect the natural flow of the blood. When this happens it causes a sudden block of the in and outflow of blood from the heart; in most cases causing heart attacks, sometimes fatal.

2. One-fourth (25%) of cholesterol comes from food intake (external source), and this is where you must be vigilant on what to take in your daily diet. Fats originated from animals are rich in cholesterol, like egg yolk, dairy, and meats, regardless of meat source. Diet plays an important part in maintaining a healthy balance.

Coronary heart disease is the leading cause of death among people living in industrialized societies such as the United States. The increasing incidence of high cholesterol levels in people residing in this part of the world can often be contributed to a high saturated fat diet, smoking and leading a sedentary lifestyle.

In 1951, a study was conducted by the US Government to find out about the importance of cholesterol and the impact it has on our health.

Pathologists were sent to Korea to examine the bodies of servicemen who lost their lives during the Korean War. Autopsies were conducted on 2,000 soldiers.

Their findings were shocking to the medical community. More than 75 percent of the soldier had yellow deposits of atherosclerotic plaque on their artery walls. With the average soldier begin 21 in age, this contradicted the assumption that artery deposits were only prevalent in older men. Before these autopsies performed during this study, doctors had no idea how early the degeneration of heart disease began.

It wasn't long after this discovery that a name was given to the major contributor to the buildup of plaque and to this heart disease risk – cholesterol.

The good news is that more recent studies have shown that for every one percent drop in cholesterol levels, there is a two percent decrease in the risk of a heart attack.

Since those original research findings, the risk of heart disease stemming from cholesterol has exploded. In 2002, it was estimated that 107 million American adults now have a blood cholesterol level high enough to require medical treatment. Unfortunately, the number of people with this condition keeps rising.

Despite this epidemic problem, there is good news. If you suffer from high cholesterol, you will find this guide filled with simple solutions for this problem. In the next few pages, we'll explore cholesterol in layman's terms, the causes, effects and what you can do to reverse the negative impact it has on your health.

How to Lower Cholesterol with Essential Oil

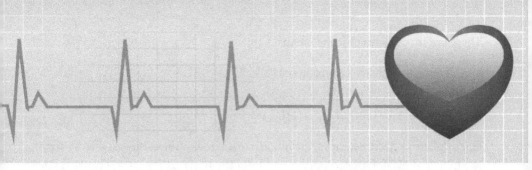

WHAT IS CHOLESTEROL?

As stated earlier, cholesterol in and of itself is a natural function of the human body. By definition, cholesterol is a waxy, fat-like substance that presents itself naturally in cell walls and membranes everywhere in your body.

Every living being requires a certain amount of fat to exist.

Your body uses cholesterol to produce many hormones. It also uses it to produce vitamin D and the bile acids that help to digest fat.

The processing of fat begins when it gets absorbed in the intestines. From there it heads to the liver. The fat requires a delivery system to the rest of the body so that it can be used immediately as well as stored in fat cells for future use.

In order for the fat to enter the delivery system, while it is in the liver it is split into two different types of fat, cholesterol, and triglycerides.

Once this transformation takes place, the two types of fat (cholesterol and triglycerides) are packed into vehicles called lipoproteins for carrying the fat to the fat cells throughout the body via the bloodstream.

There are three types of lipoproteins:

- Very Low-Density Lipoproteins (VLDL)
- Low-Density Lipoproteins (LDL)
- High-Density Lipoproteins (HDL)

Under normal circumstances, the bloodstream does a very efficient job of carrying the LDL and HDL Lipoproteins throughout the body. These packages are made of fat (lipid) on the inside and proteins on the outside. Having healthy levels of both types of lipoproteins is important.

LDL cholesterol is often referred to as "bad" cholesterol. A high LDL level leads to a buildup of cholesterol in your arteries. (Arteries are blood vessels that carry blood from your heart to your body.)

HDL cholesterol sometimes is called "good" cholesterol. This is because it carries cholesterol from other parts of your body back to your liver. Your liver is responsible for removing the cholesterol from your body.

> *Like everything in nature, it only becomes a problem when there is an imbalance.*

Problems arise when there is an overabundance of cholesterol in your bloodstream. The cholesterol deposited by the LDL leads to a narrowing of the blood vessels.

When this occurs, excess LDL cholesterol deposited in the arteries of the heart could result in a stroke or cardiovascular disease. This is called atherosclerosis. This is why LDL is known as "bad cholesterol."

> *High blood cholesterol is a condition in which you have too much cholesterol in your blood. By itself, the condition usually has no signs or symptoms. Thus, many people don't know that their cholesterol levels are too high.*

People who have high blood cholesterol have a greater chance of getting coronary heart disease, also called coronary artery disease. The higher the level of LDL cholesterol in your blood, the GREATER your risk of developing heart disease. According to the National Heart, Lung, and Blood Institute the higher the level of HDL cholesterol in your blood, the LOWER your chance is of getting heart disease.

Lowering your cholesterol may slow, reduce, or even stop the buildup of plaque in your arteries. It also may reduce the risk of plaque rupturing and cause dangerous blood clots. – NHLBI, NIH

How to Lower Cholesterol with Essential Oil

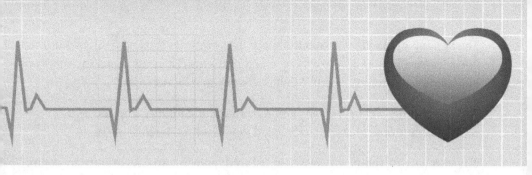

HOW CHOLESTEROL CONTRIBUTES TO HEART DISEASE

Cholesterol is not the only cause of heart disease, but it is a contributing factor. Here's how it works.

Cholesterol can only attach to the inner lining of the artery if it has been damaged.

Once the lining of the artery is damaged, white blood cells rush to the site followed by cholesterol, calcium and cellular debris. The muscle cells around the artery are altered and accumulate cholesterol.

The fatty streaks in the arteries continue to develop and bulge in the arteries. This cholesterol "bulge" is then covered by a scar that produces a hard coat or shell over the cholesterol and cell mixture. It is this collection of cholesterol that is then covered by a scar that is called "plaque."

The buildup of plaque narrows the space in the arteries through which blood can flow, decreasing the supply of oxygen and nutrients. This cuts down the supply of blood and oxygen to the tissues that are fed by that blood vessel.

> *Over time, plaque hardens and narrows your coronary arteries. This limits the flow of oxygen-rich blood to the heart. – NHLBI, NIH*

The elasticity of the blood vessel is reduced, and the arteries' ability to control blood pressure is compromised. If there is not enough oxygen-carrying blood passing through the narrowed arteries, the heart may feel compressed causing pain called angina.

> *Angina is chest pain or discomfort. It may feel like pressure or squeezing in your chest. The pain also may occur in your shoulders, arms, neck, jaw, or back. Angina pain may even feel like indigestion. – NHLBI, NIH*

The pain usually happens when you exercise because at that time your heart requires more oxygen. Often, it is felt in the chest or the left arm and shoulder, although it can happen without any symptoms at all.

> *Over time plaque can rupture (break open), causing a blood clot to form on the surface of the plaque. If the clot becomes large enough, it can mostly or completely block blood flow through a coronary artery.*

> *If the flow of oxygen-rich blood to your heart muscle is reduced or blocked, angina or heart attack may occur.*

Plaque can vary in size as well as shape. All through the coronary arteries, you can find many small plaques that cover less than half of an artery opening. Some of these plaques are completely invisible in the tests that doctors use to identify heart disease.

> *Coronary heart disease is a condition in which plaque builds up inside the coronary (heart) arteries. Plaque is made up of cholesterol, fat, calcium, and other substances found in the blood. When plaque builds up in the arteries, the condition is called atherosclerosis. – NHLBI, NIH*

The medical community used to think that the primary concern was the larger plaques, due to their size and was more likely to cause a complete blockage of the coronary arteries.

While it is true that the larger plaques are more likely to cause angina, it is the smaller plaques that are packed with cholesterol and covered by scars that are more dangerous. They are considered unstable and prone to ruptures or bursting, releasing their load of cholesterol into the bloodstream. This causes immediate clotting within the artery. If the blood clot blocks the artery entirely, it will stop the blood flow, and a heart attack occurs.

The muscle on the farther side of the occurring clot fails to get the oxygen it needs and begins to die. This kind of damage can be permanent.

A heart attack occurs if the flow of oxygen-rich blood to a section of heart muscle is cut off. If blood flow isn't restored quickly, the section of heart muscle begins to die. Without quick treatment, a heart attack can lead to serious problems or death. – NHLBI, NIH

How to Lower Cholesterol with Essential Oil

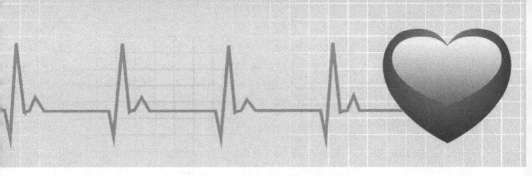

HOW DO YOU DIAGNOSE PROBLEMS WITH YOUR CHOLESTEROL?

Unfortunately, most people aren't even aware they have atherosclerosis until they have a heart attack or stroke. It is possible to have up to 80 percent closure of the arteries without ever feeling a single symptom!

Many people begin to develop cholesterol-driven atherosclerosis as children. It would be quite unusual to find an adult in the United States who does not have some degree of atherosclerosis.

Diagnosing cholesterol levels require a simple blood test to determine the levels of LDL and HDL. Cholesterol tests can be tricky, however.

In most cases, blood is drawn from a vein located on the inside of the elbow or the back of the hand. You may only have your total cholesterol level measured as the first test. This test may include measurement of your HDL cholesterol levels. If they find your cholesterol is in the normal range, you may not need additional cholesterol tests run.

Simple screening that is done without "fasting," measures only the total cholesterol and the HDL, the "good" cholesterol. The results will give you a ballpark figure, but far from accurate.

The complete test sometimes referred to as a "lipid profile," measures total cholesterol, HDL, LDL, and triglycerides. People who also have high triglyceride levels may get a test called a direct VLDL cholesterol (direct VLDL-C). Other blood tests, such as C-reactive protein (CRP), may be added to the profile in some labs.

For truly accurate numbers, you should not eat, or drink anything other than water for 12 hours before testing. Vigorous exercise should be avoided for 24 hours before testing, and you need to make certain that whoever tests you is informed of any medications you may be taking as they will also affect the results.

Your test results will come in with three numbers:

- HDL Cholesterol
- LDL Cholesterol
- Total Cholesterol

Three terms, blood cholesterol, serum cholesterol and total cholesterol all mean the same thing – the total cholesterol in your body.

For the total cholesterol, the National Cholesterol Education Program classifies levels below 200 milligrams/dl (milligrams per deciliter) as "desirable."

A level between 200 and 239 is "borderline high."

Anything over 240 is "high."

Triglyceride levels over 400 milligrams/dl are considered "high" and levels over 1,000 milligrams/dl are considered "very high."

For LDL, the desirable level is less than 130 milligrams/dl. The "borderline high" level is 130 to 159. The "high risk" level is 160 and above.

Higher is better for HDL. For HDL, the numbers are lower because there is less HDL in the blood. Anything lower than 35 milligrams/dl is considered "high risk." If your HDL is very high, say over 60, your risk of heart disease is reduced.

The LDL, however, is the "bad" cholesterol and the most important factor in predicting a heart attack. For LDL, lower is better preferably less than 160. It's best to keep the level around 130.

According to Dr. Mercola, the total cholesterol level is worthless in determining your risk for heart disease though, unless it is above 330. In an online article entitled, *The Cholesterol Myth That Could Be Harming Your Health*, he states the HDL percentage is a very potent heart disease risk factor. Just divide your HDL level by your cholesterol. That percentage should ideally be above 24 percent. You can also do the same thing with your triglycerides and HDL ratio. That percentage should be below 2.

Bear in mind, these are simply guidelines, and several other factors play into your risk of heart disease besides any of these numbers.

Dietary cholesterol means the cholesterol that you eat.

Most American food and supplement companies list cholesterol on their labels under Nutrition Facts. The American Heart Association (AHA) recommends no more than 300 milligrams per day and recommends that a triglyceride level of 100 mg/dL or lower is considered "optimal." (Cholesterol levels are measured in milligrams (mg) of cholesterol per deciliter (dL) of blood in the United States and some other countries.

TOTAL CHOLESTEROL

Below 200 mg/dL	Desirable
200-239 mg/dL	Borderline high
240 mg/dL and above	High

LDL CHOLESTEROL

Below 70 mg/dL	Ideal for people at very high risk of heart disease
Below 100 mg/dL	Ideal for people at risk of heart disease
100-129 mg/dL	Near ideal
130-159 mg/dL	Borderline high
160-189 mg/dL	High
190 mg/dL and above	Very high

HDL CHOLESTEROL

Below 40 mg/dL (men), Below 50 mg/dL (women)	Poor
50-59 mg/dL	Better
60 mg/dL and above	Best

TRIGLYCERIDES

Below 150 mg/dL	Desirable
150-199 mg/dL	Borderline high
200-499 mg/dL	High
500 mg/dL and above	Very high

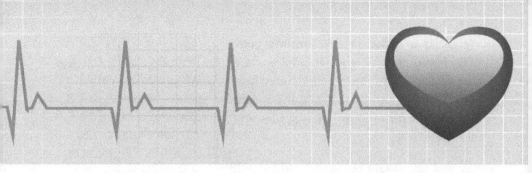

CAUSES OF
HIGH CHOLESTEROL

Earlier it was stated that Cholesterol could only attach itself to the inner lining of the artery if it has been damaged. How does that damage occur?

Evidence points to "free radical" damage as being one of the culprits of arterial wall damage. Free radicals are found all around us. They are highly reactive substances like polluted air, radiation, tobacco smoke, herbicides, and naturally within our bodies as an offshoot of normal metabolic processes.

Free radicals attack and damage cells altering normal cell activity. You see it around you every day causing the metal to rust and fruit to spoil. This is why we take anti-oxidants like vitamins C, E, beta-carotene and selenium to combat the attack of free radicals.

Heredity plays a role in high cholesterol. Your genes can influence your LDL by affecting how fast it is made and removed from your blood. There is one particular form of inherited high cholesterol that will often lead to early heart disease. It is called familial "hypercholesterolemia" and can play a role in 1 of 500 people.

Weight is a factor in determining your LDL. If you have a high LDL level and are overweight, losing those pounds may help you to lower it. Additionally, losing weight also contributes to lower triglycerides and raise your HDL.

Age and sex should be considered as well. Women, before menopause, usually have total cholesterol levels that are lower than men. This changes as men and women age. Levels will rise until reaching age 60 to 65. For women, menopause can cause an increase in LDL and a decrease in HDL. After the age of 50 women often have higher total cholesterol levels than men of the same age.

There are usually no signs or symptoms that you have high blood cholesterol, but it can be detected with a blood test. You are likely to have high cholesterol if members of your family have it, if you are overweight or if you eat a lot of fatty foods.

Alcohol plays a unique role in cholesterol levels. It increases HDL, but at the same time, it does not lower LDL. The medical community does not know for certain whether alcohol reduces the risk of heart disease. Studies do confirm too much alcohol can damage the liver and heart muscle, lead to high blood pressure and raise triglycerides. There are just too many other risks to even consider the use of alcoholic beverages as a way to prevent heart disease, just because it increases the HDL.

Stress and personality may contribute to heart disease. Associating a certain type of personality and heart disease has been suggested for many years. This goes back to the "Type A" and "Type B" personality study conducted in 1959.

Type A behavior manifests in a chronic sense of time, urgency, aggressiveness and striving for achievement. Type A people will drive themselves to meet specific deadlines which are most often self-imposed.

They have feelings of being constantly under pressure and often multitask to the point of doing two or three things at one time. To say that Type A people are "driven" is an understatement. They consider themselves indispensable. All of these traits add up to a state of constant stress.

Over the long term, stress has shown to raise blood cholesterol levels. The way it does this is by affecting habits. An example is overindulging in fatty foods as a way of consoling themselves when people are under stress. The saturated fat and cholesterol in these foods contribute to high levels of blood cholesterol. An explanation of dietary factors will be discussed in a later chapter.

Type B behavior is characterized by just the opposite set of traits. Type B people are less preoccupied with achievement, less rushed and more easygoing people.

They don't allow themselves to be rushed nor have any particular pressure regarding deadlines. They are less prone to angry outbursts and seem to be better equipped to making distinctions between work and play.

Studies completed over a period of eighteen months to two years with a group of both Type A and Type B people indicated that Type A participants had a 31 percent increased risk of developing heart disease.

This was further substantiated by the discovery of more deposits of plaque in the coronary arteries of Type A people. Type A behavior also appears to show an association with other risk factors like smoking, higher fat levels, increased secretion of adrenaline. All of which increases the oxygen requirement of the heart muscles and releasing fatty acids from the body fat.

While each person may not fall into one distinct category, it is important to understand that every person is unique and what lifestyle changes need to be made will vary from each individual, and health care regimens will depend on their lifestyle and particular needs.

How to Lower Cholesterol with Essential Oil

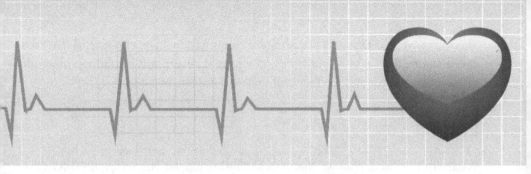

PRESCRIBED MEDICATIONS FOR CHOLESTEROL

Many of those reading this book may already be taking several medications for controlling cholesterol. In this chapter, the different types of medications will be covered. Your doctor may decide that you need help in controlling your cholesterol if you are unable to reduce it using natural methods.

> "If you are concerned about your cholesterol levels, taking a drug should be your absolute last resort. And when I say last resort, I'm saying the odds are very high, greater than 100 to 1, that you don't need drugs to lower your cholesterol." – Dr. Joseph Mercola

Even if your doctor prescribes any of these medications, you must still follow through with healthy lifestyle treatments that will be discussed later on.

There are several different types of medications used to lower cholesterol. They are called statins, bile acid sequestrants, cholesterol absorption inhibitors, nicotinic acid agents, and fibrates, and we will review them one by one.

STATINS

What are they and how do they work? Statins repress the enzyme HMG-CoA reductase. This enzyme controls the rate that cholesterol produces itself in the body. These drugs can lower cholesterol from 20 to 60%. They slow the production while they increase the liver's ability to withdraw LDL. Statins lower the LDL levels better than any other type of drug.

They can also produce a modest increase of HDL while decreasing total cholesterol and triglycerides. Positive results are usually seen after just 4 to 6 weeks of beginning the medication.

Overall statins are proven for lowering heart attack risks, strokes and other coronary diseases related to high cholesterol levels. You should not take statins if:

- You are allergic to statins themselves or their ingredients
- You are pregnant or breastfeeding
- You have liver disease
- You consume excessive amounts of alcohol
- Have a history of myopathy
- Have renal failure

Brand names of statins that you might recognize are Lipitor, Lescol, Mevacor, Altocor, Pravachol, Zocor, and Crestor.

There are some drug and food interactions that you should be aware of. More than one quart of grapefruit juice per day can decrease the ability of the liver to process some statins. More importantly, there may be other medications that can interact and cause serious side effects. It's important to let your doctor know about any other medication you are taking, whether prescription or non-prescription including vitamins, herbal supplements, medication for the immune system, other cholesterols drugs, medication for infections, birth control pills, medication for heart failure, HIV or AIDs, or Coumadin.

Side effects from statins are rare. If you experience muscle soreness, pain, weakness, vomiting, stomach pain, discolored urine, stop taking the medication and contact your doctor immediately.

BILE ACID SEQUESTRANTS

Bile acid sequestrants bind with bile acids that contain cholesterol in the intestines and are then eliminated in the stool. They are proven to reduce LDL by 10 to 20%. Small doses produce decent reductions in LDL. They are sometimes prescribed along with a statin to enhance reduction. When combined, their effects are counted together and lower LDL by more than 40%. They do not lower triglycerides.

People who are allergic to bile acid sequestrants should not take this medication nor should anyone who has a medical history of bile obstruction.

There may be interactions with other drugs so make certain your doctor has a complete list of all prescribed and non-prescribed medications you are taking.

Bile acid sequestrants do not become absorbed from the gastrointestinal tract. It has been used for 30+ years and is considered safe for long term use.

CHOLESTEROL ABSORPTION INHIBITORS

A newer drug class, Zetia is a cholesterol absorption inhibitor that was approved in 2002 by the FDA. By itself, it reduces LDL by 18 to 20%. It does this by decreasing absorption of cholesterol and other drugs within this class also mildly lower triglycerides.

Very useful for prescribing to people who cannot take statins or as another drug that can be taken if those who take statins have side effects if the statin dose is increased. Adding a cholesterol inhibitor to a statin increased the lowering effect by a 2 to 3 fold factor.

There may be interactions with other drugs so make certain your doctor has a complete list of all prescribed and non-prescribed medications you are taking.

NICOTINIC ACID AGENTS

Niacin, Niacor, and Slo-Niacin are common names for nicotinic acid agents.

Nicotinic acid, which is also called niacin, is a water-soluble vitamin B. It improves levels of all lipoproteins when the doses are given far above the vitamin requirement.

Nicotinic acid reduces total cholesterol, LDL, and triglycerides at the same time raising HDL. It reduces LDL by 10 to 20%, triglycerides by 20 to 50% and increases HDL by 15 to 35%. Nicotinamide is a niacin by-product after the body breaks it down. Nicotinamide has no effect in lowering cholesterol and should not be used in place of nicotinic acid.

Individuals who are allergic to nicotinic acid, and those who have liver disease, active peptic ulcer, or arterial bleeding, should not use nicotinic acid agents.

There are two types of nicotinic acid. One for immediate release and one for extended release. Immediate release is inexpensive and widely available without a prescription. However, because of potential side effects, it must not be used for lowering cholesterol without being monitored by a doctor.

Niacin that is extended release is often tolerated better than crystalline niacin. But has a greater chance of causing damage to the liver.

If you are taking medication for high blood pressure, the results may be increased while taking niacin. You should have a system available to monitor your blood pressure when beginning a new niacin regimen.

Again, there may be side effects when mixed with other medications or foods. Discuss with your doctor and make certain you make him aware of all medications prescribed or otherwise.

FIBRATES

Primary effectiveness is lowering triglycerides. There is a lesser effect in increasing HDL levels.

Some serious side effects may occur so be sure and discuss these with your doctor. If you are allergic to fibrates or have liver disease or kidney disease, you should not take these agents. All adults should have their blood pressure checked annually if their blood pressure was less than 120/80 mmHg at their last reading. If you have high blood pressure, diabetes, kidney problems, or another health condition, you will want to have your high blood pressure checked more often. Your health care provider will measure your blood pressure several times before diagnosing you with high blood pressure. It is normal for your blood pressure to vary at different times a day. Readings performed at home with proper equipment will give you a more accurate reading of your current blood pressure than one taken at a grocery store, a fire station or doctor's office.

> *"Conventional medicine misses the boat entirely when they dangerously recommend that lowering cholesterol with drugs is the way to reduce your risk of heart attacks because what is actually needed is to address whatever is causing your body damage -- and leading to increased inflammation and then increased cholesterol." – Dr. Joseph Mercola*

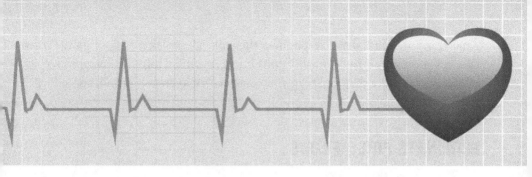

NATURAL TREATMENTS

No medications can do a better job than treating your high cholesterol naturally. And, if you are one of those lucky people who does not have cholesterol concerns, you may want to take steps to keep it that way!

What can you do to improve your cholesterol levels? Here's the list and we will cover each item thoroughly.

REDUCE FAT IN YOUR DIET

One of the best plans is covered previously in our chart on saturated fat. But there is more you can do. Buy the leanest cuts of meat you can find. Regularly substitute poultry (without the skin) and fish for red meat. Both are lower in saturated fat. Switch to low-fat cottage cheese and yogurt, reduced fat hard cheeses and skim or 1 percent milk.

EAT NO MORE THAN FOUR EGG YOLKS A WEEK

Many people don't have to worry about eating cholesterol. Normal bodies adjust to increased intake by cutting back on the product. However, since one-third of

Americans are cholesterol responders their blood cholesterol does go up when they eat cholesterol. You probably don't know if you fall into this category so play it safe. Eat no more than four egg yolks a week. An average egg yolk contains 213 milligrams of cholesterol!

ELIMINATE FRIED FOODS

Buying low fat is just the beginning. You need to institute low-fat cooking methods to keep the cholesterol from sneaking back into your diet.

- Remove fatty skin from chicken and turkey.
- Don't fry foods. Roast, bake, broil, grill or poach them instead.
- Use fat-free marinades or basting with liquids like wine, tomato or lemon juice.
- Use olive or canola oils for sautéing or baking. Both are very low in saturated fat.
- Use diet, tub or squeeze margarine instead of regular. Watch for the term "hydrogenated," which means some of the fat is saturated.

EAT VEGETABLES AND COMPLEX CARBOHYDRATES

Lowest fat foods of all are vegetables, fruits, grains (rice, barley, and pasta), beans and legumes. Try substituting some of these for meat and high-fat dairy products.

- Don't douse your pasta with butter or your potato with sour cream.
- Use tomato based sauces instead of cream base.
- Use lemon juice, low sodium soy sauce or herbs to season vegetables.
- Make chili with extra beans and seasonings while leaving out the meat.

Improve eating habits by eating rich high-fiber foods including oatmeal or bran. Be sure to include fish and omega-3 fatty acids, walnuts, almonds, and other nuts. Substitute fats with olive oil. Check for foods that contain a natural additive called sterols (or stanols) that are beneficial.

LOSE WEIGHT

If you are overweight, the chances are almost 100% that you have a problem with high cholesterol. You can lower your LDL and elevate your HDL just by dropping some pounds. Eat fewer fatty foods and more fruits, vegetables, grains, and beans, and it's a pretty good bet that you will gradually lose weight.

INCLUDE YOUR FAMILY

Eating habits carry through to adulthood. Get your children on a healthy eating pattern early. Don't begin until they are at least two years of age, however. Babies need extra fat calories to develop properly.

SNACK ALL YOU WANT

Snack several times a day on low-fat foods. Yogurt, fruit, vegetables, bagels and whole grain breads and cereals are excellent for snacking. In fact, there is evidence that points to lower cholesterol levels in people who eat several small meals a day. Eating often can keep hormones like insulin from rising and signaling your body to make more cholesterol. Make certain that your total intake of calories doesn't go up when you eat more often.

GO NUTS

Do you like nuts? If you do, sprinkle a few on your cereal, bake them into muffins or pancakes or add them to casseroles or stir-fries. Walnuts and almonds are especially good. Eating about three ounces of walnuts a day is shown to decrease blood cholesterol levels by 10% more than an already low fat, low cholesterol diet. Walnuts are high in fat, but it is mostly polyunsaturated fat, which is the kind that lowers cholesterol. Another study shows that about three ounces of almonds which are rich in monounsaturated fat lower LDL by 9%.

EAT CHOCOLATE

Aha! All you chocoholics rejoice! Studies indicate that the fat in chocolate is stearic acid and has no effect on cholesterol levels. The chocolate does not increase LDL and could raise HDL a wee bit. But chocolate is still high in fat and calories so don't go overboard.

DRINK FRUIT JUICES

You may have read about the low rate of heart disease in France. It led researchers to believe that the French habit of drinking red wine with meals contributes to this. Apparently, some of the non-alcoholic ingredients in red wine raise HDL and suppress the body from producing LDL.

Purple grape juice works the same way. It will work like red wine to lower the fat level in your blood. The LDL-lowering effect of red wine and grape juice comes from a compound that grapes normally produce to resist mold. The darker the grape juice, the better.

Grapefruit juice does the same thing, and it may also help your body get rid of that nasty plaque that we discussed earlier.

EAT GARLIC

Cholesterol-lowering effects of garlic have repeatedly been demonstrated in people with healthy and high cholesterol. Eat all the garlic you can. It also seems to raise the HDL levels as well. If you are worried about the odor, take the tablets instead. They have proven to be nearly as effective as the cooked or raw cloves.

TAKE NIACIN – CAREFULLY

We discussed niacin earlier. Remember as one of the B vitamins; it is proven effective for lowering LDL and raising HDL. It is also one of the cheapest drugs available for lowering cholesterol. But, without medical supervision, it may not be safe. A dose high enough to lower cholesterol can cause extremely high blood sugar or liver damage.

TAKE VITAMIN E

Studies indicate that vitamin E may have a positive impact on lowering cholesterol when taken in relatively large quantities – up to 800 IU per day. This is more than you can get from your diet alone. More Copious amounts do not seem to cause any harm. Further studies showed that even amounts of just 25 IU per day help in preventing LDL from sticking to blood vessel walls. That amount is only slightly higher than the recommended daily amount (RDA) of 12 to 15 IU. It's interesting to note that even that small amount has an impact on preventing that hardening of the arteries.

TAKE CALCIUM

One study indicates that when 56 people took a calcium carbonate supplement, their total cholesterol went down 4 percent and their HDL increased 4 percent. That was taking a dosage of 400 milligrams of calcium three times a day with no harmful effects reported. That does refer to calcium carbonate.

TAKE A MULTIVITAMIN

While you are building your calcium and vitamin E intake, remember the old standby, vitamin C. It is the number one immune system booster and also drives up HDL. A study of people who took more than 60 milligrams of vitamin C per day (60 milligrams is the RDA) had highest LDL levels.

FILL UP ON FIBER

Remember several years back when oat bran was the latest craze for lowering cholesterol? Later studies arrived at inconsistent results, but the medical community does agree that soluble fiber, the kind found in oat bran, does help lower LDL and raise HDL. As little as three grams per day of fiber from oat bran or oatmeal can be effective. There are 7.2 grams of soluble fiber per 100 grams of dry oat bran and five grams of soluble fiber per 100 grams of dry oatmeal. There are other sources of fiber as well such as barley, beans, peas and many other vegetables. Corn fiber is also good for reducing LDL, lowering it by as much as 5 percent in a recent study. Researchers used 20 grams of corn fiber a day. That would be a bit difficult for the average user when you take into account that one serving of corn has three grams of corn fiber. But, every little bit does make a difference. Pectin, which is found in fruits like apples and prunes, reduces cholesterol even better than oat bran, as does psyllium which is the fiber you find in many breakfast cereals and bulk laxatives.

QUIT SMOKING

Smoking promotes the development of atherosclerosis. Tobacco smoke is more damaging to the heart than the lungs. Smokers have a higher chance of having a heart attack (three times greater than nonsmokers) and an increased risk of dying from an attack (twenty-one times higher than nonsmokers.) Tobacco smoke contains carbon monoxide, which is uniquely damaging to the heart.

Not only does it reduce the amount of oxygen the heart receives, but it also actually damages the cells of the heart, rendering them less able to produce energy and thereby weakening the heart. In addition to the dangers of carbon monoxide, there's the risk of the nicotine. Nicotine interferes with the electrical impulses that cause the heart to beat. When the blood flow is compromised, the heart can beat in a fast, uncontrolled, irregular beats that actually cause a heart attack. If you smoke, reducing the risks of atherosclerosis is yet another reason to stop. Even if you have smoked for years, stopping now can still immediately help combat the development of atherosclerosis.

REDUCE SUGAR INTAKE

Many people don't realize that sugar affects cholesterol and triglycerides. Sugar stimulates insulin production, which in turn increases triglycerides. Men, in particular, seem to be sensitive to this effect from sugar. The mineral chromium which helps to stabilize blood sugar can also raise the level of HDL. 100 mcg of chromium three times daily can contribute to improving your cholesterol levels.

ELIMINATE ALCOHOL

The jury is still out, and the different schools of thought are still at odds regarding the benefit or lack of benefit to consuming alcohol. This suggestion has nothing to do with our previous discussion on red wine. A moderate amount may be helpful. The problem is that to one person a reasonable amount might be a glass of wine with their meal, while to another it might be a half bottle of Scotch! Anything above the arbitrary "moderate" amount elevates serum cholesterol triglycerides and your uric acid levels as well as potentially increasing blood pressure all of which promote heart disease. So, the best bet would be to eliminate it.

EXERCISE REGULARLY

There is conclusive evidence that exercise can lower LDL cholesterol and boost HDL cholesterol. Both aerobic exercise such as walking, jogging, swimming, bicycling and cross country skiing and strength training like lifting weights or using weight machines all promote the improvement of cholesterol levels. An analysis of 11 studies on weight training showed that this exercise lowered LDL by 13 percent and raised HDL by 5 percent. If you lift weights, use light to moderate weights and do many repetitions.

ELIMINATE CAFFEINE

Americans have a love affair with coffee. People who drink significant amounts of caffeine (more than 6 cups a day) are far more prone to elevated cholesterol. That connection does not hold for tea drinkers. Limit your coffee intake to no more than one cup a day and eliminate caffeinated sodas entirely.

HERBAL REMEDIES

Unfortunately, the medical community is quick to prescribe another expensive medication to lower cholesterol, but they are far less likely to suggest herbal or homeopathic measures.

Along with getting plenty of fiber, some foods will help in promoting the lowering of cholesterol as well as herbs that can further reduce cholesterol.

Foods containing pectin are advantageous to lowering cholesterol levels. Carrots, apples and the white layer inside of citrus rinds are particularly beneficial.

Avocado, which is very high in fat, has unexpectedly become a cholesterol reducer. A study of women who were given a choice of a high monounsaturated fat (olive oil) along with avocado diet or a complex carbohydrate consisting of starches and sugars reported impressive results. In six weeks, the former group on the olive oil and avocado diet showed an 8.2 percent reduction in cholesterol.

Beans. Have to love them. They are high in fiber and low in cholesterol. What more could you ask for! A cup and a half of beans, or the amount in a bowl of soup, can lower total cholesterol levels by as much as 19 percent!

Garlic. We discussed garlic earlier, but it is well worth repeating here. Use it liberally in your diet. Not only will it help to lower your cholesterol it is also credited with lowering blood pressure. Be sure you include generous amounts of garlic as well as onions in your daily diet.

Cayenne pepper (Capsicum minimum) and other plants that contain the phenolic compound capsaicin have a well-demonstrated effect in lowering blood cholesterol levels, as does the widely used spice Fenugreek.

Caraway is another aromatic spice with demonstrable cholesterol lowering properties.

A whole range of Asian herbal remedies new to western medicine is proving to be valuable in this field.

If you have cholesterol concerns and cannot change the way you eat, there is still an option that is nearly as effective as statin drugs. People with total cholesterol levels slightly above 200 should consider adding plenty of foods with phytosterols to their current diet. These compounds decrease the amount of cholesterol that is absorbed into the bloodstream and can be found in:

- Sunflower seeds
- Corn
- Pure tall oil (or liquid rosin) [4]
- Flaxseed
- Rye bread
- Almonds
- Broccoli
- Carrots
- Spinach
- Strawberries
- Blueberries

The more phytosterols that are consumed, the less cholesterol enters the blood. Two to three servings per day have been shown to reduce total cholesterol by 10% and LDL by 14%. The phytosterols themselves are not absorbed, so there are no side effects. Source: https://www.ncbi.nlm.nih.gov/pubmed/12963571

Remember when the "low-fat" mantra began? We all jumped in with both feet, and some of us still live on low-fat foods, like having a baked potato with no butter or sour cream. Maybe you eat pasta, veggies, and fat-free desserts. So how come you still gain weight?

Good question. Researchers from the National Center for Health Statistics studied the eating habits of 8.260 adult Americans between 1988 and 1991. They found that Americans have significantly reduced their fat intake but still packed on extra pounds in recent years.

In fact, a national health and nutrition survey of over 8,000 American adults concludes that one-third of the population is overweight.

Experts suggest taking cholesterol-lowering supplements such as artichoke extract, barley, beta-sitosterol, blond psyllium (found in seed husk and products such as Metamucil), fish oil (found as a liquid oil and in oil-filled capsules), flaxseed, garlic extract, green tea extract, oat bran, stanols, and red yeast rice.

The answer is straightforward and right in front of us. So many of us jumped on the low-fat diet and assumed that if it's low fat, it can't make us fat. Right? Wrong. We were so involved with the low-fat concept that we forgot to count calories!

If you are eating more calories than your body needs, whether, from fat or carbohydrates, the body will store them as fat. Period. According to a National Institutes of Health study, by 1990 the average American was consuming hundreds of more calories a day than he was consuming ten years before.

Some researchers believe that eating small amounts of fat can keep you from overindulging on total calories. Ohio State University nutrition scientist John Allred points out that dietary fat causes our bodies to produce a hormone that tells our intestines to slow down the emptying process. We feel full and are less likely to overeat.

Add a little bit of peanut butter to your piece of fruit, and it can help to keep you from a binge later.

Here is another trap to avoid. Reducing fat might not be as smart as it sounds. Tufts University scientists recently placed 11 middle-aged men and women volunteers on a variety of healthy reduced and low-fat diets.

The results were astounding. Very low-fat diets which provided only 15 percent of fat from calories did have a positive effect on blood cholesterol and triglyceride levels. By the way, that diet is so strict there is no way it could be duplicated in real life. But a reduced fat diet, which is more realistic, only affected those levels if accompanied by weight loss.

Not only that, they concluded that cutting fat without losing weight increased triglyceride levels and decreased HDL.

So while excess fat is not healthy, it isn't a dirty word either. Without some fat in our diets, our bodies could not make nerve cells and hormones or absorb fat soluble vitamins.

If obesity is one of your high cholesterol causes, try losing a pound a week with a 500 calorie solution. No, we aren't going to ask you only to eat 500 calories a week!

What you can do is easily lose a pound a week just by cutting 500 calories a day out of your diet. You can easily burn 250 of them just be spending about 30 minutes of aerobic exercise, like bicycling, dancing or just walking. To get rid of the other 250 try cutting out mayonnaise, doughnuts, and alcohol.

If there were no other reason to take control of cholesterol, here's one that certainly has merit.

A recent study found that men with high cholesterol are twice as likely to be impotent as men whose cholesterol levels are normal or low.

Researchers recorded cholesterol levels of 3,250 healthy men between the ages of 25 and 83. Men with total cholesterol higher than 240 milligrams/dl were twice as likely to have trouble achieving or maintaining an erection than men who cholesterol levels were below 180 milligrams/dl.

Men who had low levels of HDL were also twice as likely to suffer from impotence. The same high-fat diet that narrows arteries and blocks blood flow to your heart also narrows the arteries that carry blood to your penis. Blood has to be able to get to your penis for you to have an erection. Take control now, and you'll find yourself improving in this area of your life as well.

The typical American diet consists of fatty meats, processed cold cuts, dairy products, and fried foods. As if that weren't enough, throw in commercially baked breads, rolls, cakes, chips, and cookies. This is a surefire path to high cholesterol.

Oddly, ingesting cholesterol will not raise the blood cholesterol nearly as much as eating a type of fat called "saturated fat." Like cholesterol, saturated fat is primarily found in animal products like cheese, butter, cream, whole milk, ice cream, lard and marbled meats.

Don't believe that if you just change to vegetable oil, you can eliminate the problem. Some vegetable oils are also high in saturated fat. Palm oil, palm kernel oil, coconut oil and cocoa butter are also very high in saturated fat. Unfortunately, these are also most often used in commercially baked goods, coffee creams, and nondairy whipped toppings, so make sure you read labels. Canola oil (7% saturated fat) is one of the best available cooking oils. Olive oil (14% saturated fat) is also good to use.

Trans fatty acids may be as bad for you as saturated fat, so stick margarine is equal to butter as far as your cholesterol is concerned. Diet and soft margarine are a better bet. Also look for brands of margarine or shortening that top the ingredient list with oils rich in monounsaturated fat, like canola oil.

Another option is to substitute butter and margarine with a fruit puree. Prune puree may not sound like a particularly attractive alternative, but using applesauce and apricots as substitutes may.

The only drawback to using fruits like applesauce and apricots as fat substitutes is that baked goods tend to become soggy and moldy within a day or two so plan quantities accordingly. Also, when baking with substitutes for fat, use cake flour instead of regular all-purpose flour. It will keep the baked good tender. Don't overbake your fat reduced recipes as they do tend to dry out quicker than traditional recipes that call for butter or oil.

Here's another healthy living tip for you. If you have trouble giving up your favorite high fat cheese, try this. Turn it into a low-fat version. Just zap it in the microwave for a minute or two. Pull it out and drain off the oil. It will significantly reduce the fat content of the cheese. This will work well for cheese sandwiches, toppings and other recipes that call for your favorite cheese.

Scientists have discovered that water mixed with fructose suppresses the appetite better than glucose with water or even diet drinks. Fructose is the kind of sugar found in fruits. Drink a glass of fructose-rich orange juice a half hour to an hour before a meal. You will eat fewer calories during the next meal and still feel comfortably full.

Don't think that just because we are discussing "fat-free" regimens that you must cut beef completely out of your diet. Too much of this "good thing" won't do you any favors. However, you can have your steak and eat it too, provided it's a cut that is relatively low in fat and cholesterol, and you do not add fat in the cooking and serving process.

When shopping for beef, select grade eye of the round is considered by some to be just that. A 3 ½ ounce serving has approximately four grams of fat, less than half of the amount in a 1 ounce serving of cheddar cheese. It also contains 69 milligrams of cholesterol, among 5the lowest for meats, and it is an excellent source of zinc, iron and other nutrients.

Tip round, bottom round and top sirloin are also relatively lean and high in these nutrients.

Turkey breast and chicken breast are prizes as soon as you remove the skin. Turkey has less than 1 gram of fat and 83 milligrams of cholesterol. Chicken has 3.6 grams of fat and 85 milligrams of cholesterol.

Pork tenderloin is the top choice for the "other white meat," while leg shank is the leanest choice among lamb cuts.

TIP: Research conducted at the Copenhagen University found two tablespoons of honey and three teaspoons of Cinnamon Powder (or 1-3 drops of essential oil) mixed in 16 ounces of tea water given to a cholesterol patients reduce the level of cholesterol in the blood by 10% within 2 hours.

Cinnamon has blood-thinning properties that can help lower cholesterol levels, says Vasant Lad, B.A.M.S., M.A.Sc, director of the Ayurvedic Institute in Albuquerque, New Mexico. He suggests this tea:

Mix 1 teaspoon of cinnamon and ¼ teaspoon of Trikatu (a blend of ginger and two kinds of peppers) directly into a cup of hot water, then stir and steep for five minutes. Add a teaspoon of honey once the tea has cooled.

Dr. Lad says to drink this beverage twice daily, once in the morning and once in the evening. Trikatu is available from Ayurvedic practitioners and in some health food stores.

DETOX

One way to heal many health problems is with a detoxification diet that cleanses the body and re-establishes the nutritional balance needed for optimum health, says Elson Haas, M.D., director of the Preventive Medical Center of Marin in San Rafael, California, and author of *Staying Healthy With Nutrition*. His diet should be practiced for only three weeks. It is not nutritionally balanced enough for long periods. Do not undergo it if you are pregnant or suffer from deficiency problems marked by fatigue, coldness or heart weakness.

Here is the detox diet.

BREAKFAST

Immediately upon arising, drink two glasses of water, one of them containing the juice of half of a lemon. Also have one to two servings of fresh fruit – apples, pears, bananas, grapes or citrus fruits such as oranges or grapefruit.

About 15 to 30 minutes later, have one to two cups of cooked oatmeal, brown rice millet, amaranth or untoasted buckwheat. For flavoring, you can add two tablespoons of fruit juice.

LUNCH

Have a big bowl (up to four cups) of steamed vegetables – potatoes, yams, green beans, broccoli, kale, cauliflower, carrots, beets, asparagus, cabbage or others. Use a variety, including stems, roots, and greens. Better Butter can also be used. Then refrigerate the water from the vegetables for later use.

Within two hours, slowly drink one to two cups of the water from the steamed vegetables. You can add a little sea salt or kelp for flavoring.

DINNER

Same as lunch, with a variety of vegetables.

EVENING (AFTER DINNER)

No food at all, but you can have non-caffeinated herbal teas such as peppermint, chamomile or blends. No caffeinated beverages.

Throughout the day, feelings of hunger should be satisfied by drinking plenty of water and eating pieces of carrot or celery. If you are feeling very fatigued or if hunger persists, then you may add up to four ounces of protein, such as fish, organic chicken, lentils or garbanzo, mung or black beans. Optimally this should be eaten mid-afternoon, around 3:00 or 4:00.

Again, this is a detoxification diet only and is to cleanse the body and re-establish nutritional balance needed for optimum health. Do not practice the diet for more than three weeks and do not undergo it if you are pregnant or suffer from deficiency problems.

When eating out at a restaurant, opt for steamed, grilled or broiled dishes instead of those that are fried or sautéed.

Eat more dark green veggies, such as broccoli, kale, and other dark leafy greens; orange veggies, such as carrots, sweet potatoes, pumpkin, and winter squash; and beans and peas, such as pinto beans, kidney beans, black beans, garbanzo beans, split peas, and lentils.

Read the Nutrition Facts label on foods. Look for foods low in saturated fats and trans fats. Choose and prepare foods and beverages with a little salt (sodium) and added sugars (caloric sweeteners).

If you eat 100 more food calories a day than you burn, you'll gain about 1 pound in a month. That's about 10 pounds in a year. The bottom line is that to lose weight; it's important to reduce calories and increase physical activity.

Know the facts about what you are purchasing to eat. Read labels carefully.

Most packaged foods have a Nutrition Facts label. For a healthier, you, use this tool to make smart food choices quickly and easily. Try these tips:

- Keep these low: saturated fats, trans fats, cholesterol, and sodium.
- Get enough of these: potassium, fiber, vitamins A and C, calcium, and iron.
- Use the % Daily Value (DV) column when possible: 5% DV or less is low, 20% DV or more is high.

Look at the serving size and how many servings you are consuming. If you double the servings you eat, you double the calories and nutrients, including the % DVs.

Make your calories count. Look at the calories on the label and compare them with what nutrients you are also getting to decide whether the food is worth eating. When one serving of a single food item has over 400 calories per serving, it is high in calories.

Don't sugarcoat it. Since sugars contribute calories with few, if any, nutrients, look for foods and beverages low in added sugars. Read the ingredient list and make sure that added sugars are not one of the first few ingredients. Some names for added sugars (caloric sweeteners) include sucrose, glucose, high fructose corn syrup, corn syrup, maple syrup, and fructose.

Know your fats. Look for foods low in saturated fats, trans fats, and cholesterol to help reduce the risk of heart disease (5% DV or less is low, 20% DV or more is high). Most of the fats you eat should be polyunsaturated and monounsaturated fats. Keep total fat intake between 20% to 35% of calories.

Reduce sodium (salt), increase potassium.

Research shows that eating less than 2,300 milligrams of sodium (about 1 Tsp of salt) per day may reduce the risk of high blood pressure. Most of the sodium people eat comes from processed foods, not from the salt shaker. Also look for foods high in potassium, which counteracts some of the sodium's effects on blood pressure.

Make certain that you explain any new treatments with your health care provider before embarking on any radical health changes you are anticipating.

LOWER CHOLESTEROL WITH WATER

Did you know that people who don't drink enough water have higher blood cholesterol levels? This is because the body adjusts its cholesterol distribution to protect cells from dehydration. Studies showed that when a person doesn't drink enough water in as few as 12 hours on average had 8% more total cholesterol and 5% more bad cholesterol in their blood. The good news is, levels will return to normal when the body is rehydrated. According to research, men should drink approximately 3 liters per day. Women should drink 2.2 liters per day.

(Source: http://www.naturalhealthadvisory.com/daily/cholesterol-control/how-do-you-lower-cholesterol-levels-try-these-3-simple-diet-plans/)

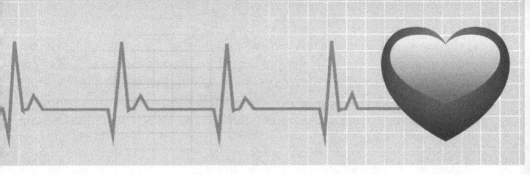

WHAT IS AN
ESSENTIAL OIL?

Before examining how essential oils can help lower cholesterol, let's first look at what an essential oil is and how it works.

Essential oils are a fragrant, vital fluid distilled from flowers, shrubs, leaves, trees, roots, and seeds. Because they are necessary for the life of the plant and play a vital role in the biological processes of the vegetation, these substances are called "essential." They carry the lifeblood, intelligence, and vibrational energy that endow them with the healing power to sustain their own life—and help the people who use them.

TIP: Before using essential oils for any health condition, be sure to study each essential oils' profile to learn how each one works in general, as well as learn about their unique characteristics.

Since essential oils are derived from a natural plant source, you will notice that the oil does not leave an "oily" or greasy spot. Unlike fatty vegetable oils used for cooking (composed of molecules too large to penetrate at a cellular level), essential oils are a non-greasy liquid composed of tiny molecules that can permeate every cell and administer healing at the most fundamental level of our body. Their unique chemical makeup allows them to pass through the skin and the cell membranes where most needed. Whether diffused into the air or applied to the skin, they immediately are absorbed and go straight to action and can perform various functions.

Modern medicine has attempted to replicate the chemical constituents and healing capabilities of essential oils, but cannot. This is because man-made pharmaceuticals lack the intelligence and life-force found in the healing oils. Most synthetic prescriptions have several undesirable side effects—even some that are detrimental.

In general, essential oils have no serious side effects that are deadly. Many people have reported authentic healing when using them—though everyone may not experience the same results as family history, lifestyle, and diet plays a significant role in the body's healing process. Essential oils work together in harmony, making them inherently safe, unlike when multiple prescription drugs are taken, causing drug-interaction.

Some of the aromatic plants and their parts in which essential oils come from include trees, grasses, fruit, leaves, flowers, bark, needles, roots, and seeds.

Also, all essential oils have unique medicinal properties, characteristics and therapeutic benefits that will differ depending on the soil, climate, and altitude of the countries where the plants were grown.

Plant substances that have been extracted into essential oils are used in aromatherapy to promote well-being and good health. While the term aromatherapy can seem ambiguous, "scent" is only one aspect of aromatherapy, as you will discover many more dramatic benefits for healing the body, mind, and spirit.

SMART TIP: You can also consume lemongrass oil by drinking lemongrass tea, made by infusing the leaves, which contain 0.4 percent essential oil, in hot water.

ESSENTIAL OILS RECOMMENDED FOR LOWERING CHOLESTEROL

The following is a list of essential oils that may help regulate cholesterol levels in the body and have a role in the prevention of atherosclerosis due to their antioxidant activity against LDL. Essential oils' chemical constituents that have therapeutic potential as dietary supplements include terpinolene, y-terpinene, eugenol, and thymol. Those oils that have been identified as LDL anti-oxidants include tea tree (terpinolene, y-terpinene), mountain pine (tepinolene), thyme (thymol), clove bud (eugenol), narcissus absolute, petitgrain, and the citrus oils such as bergamot, lemon, and lime (y-terpinene).

There are several oils to choose from; however, those that are instant favorites among essential oil enthusiasts include Lemongrass (Cymbopogon Citratus or Cymbopogon flexuous) because of its rich in geraniol and citral. Clinical aromatherapists commonly recommend it for treating circulatory conditions, by rubbing a few drops of the essential oil on the skin (diluted with a carrier oil) of the affected areas to improve and increase blood flow. It's fresh, citrusy scent is quite invigorating, loaded with antiseptic properties. Lemongrass serves as a great anti-depressant, as well as tones and fortifies the nervous system. Lemongrass is a favorite herb used in detoxifying the digestive organs of the body, like pancreas, liver, kidney, and bladder. The FDA has certified Lemongrass as GRAS (generally regarded as safe), so it may be ingested for help with cholesterol and other issues such as digestive or stomach issues, indigestion, constipation or flatulence. To use, dissolve 1-2 drops of Lemongrass in a teaspoon of honey, or place on a sugar cube, and add to a ¼ cup of water. You may also place the oil into a capsule with a base carrier oil such as coconut oil for easy ingestion as well.

TIP: Some herbalists and essential oils enthusiasts make a tea with Lemongrass drinking 1-4 cups per day to relieve health issues such as congestion, coughing, bladder infections, headaches, fever, stomach aches, digestive problems, diarrhea, bowel spasms, vomiting, flu symptoms. It also works as a mild sedative and promotes perspiration, as well as a supportive agent to help the body regulate and lower cholesterol. Lemongrass essential oil (3-4 drops) can be placed on a sugar cube for these uses as well. The leaves of lemongrass can also be dried and made into a powder for use in capsules.

The Department of Nutritional Sciences at the University of Wisconsin investigated the link between lemongrass and cholesterol and published their findings in 1989 in the medical journal, *Lipids*. In this study, they conducted a clinical trial involving 22 people with high cholesterol who took 140-mg capsules of lemongrass oil daily. While cholesterol levels were only slightly affected in some of the participants, cholesterol was lowered from 310 to 294 on average, while other people that participated in the study experienced a significant decrease in blood fats. The latter group, characterized as responders, experienced a 25-point drop in cholesterol after one month, with this positive trend continuing over the course of the short study. After three months, cholesterol levels among the responders had decreased by a significant 38 points. Interestingly, when the responders stopped taking lemongrass essential oil capsules, their cholesterol returned to previous levels. This study did not involve a placebo group, which is typically used to help measure the effects of the agent being studied.

A second favorite is Cinnamon Bark (Cinnamomum zeylanicum), which has been researched regarding its benefits for patients with diabetes. According to one report, they found that intake of 1, 3, or 6 g of cinnamon per day reduced serum glucose, triglyceride, LDL (bad) cholesterol, and the total cholesterol in people with type 2 diabetes (Diabetes Care, 2003 Dec;26(12):3215-8). Harvard Medical School recommends consuming as little as ½ teaspoon of cinnamon each day. This can reduce your blood sugar, cholesterol and triglyceride levels by as much as 12-30% ("Eat, Drink and Be Healthy: The Harvard Medical School Guide to Healthy Eating"; Walter Willett and P. J. Skerrett; 2005.). Cinnamon Bark essential oil promotes circulation and supports a healthy immune system. Cinnamon essential oil is used at a dose of 0.05 to 0.2 g daily (1 drop – 4 drops).

Ever wonder why your mom always adds a bay leaf to the spaghetti sauce or pot of soup? In a 2009 study in the "Journal of Clinical Biochemistry and Nutrition," they reported on the effects bay leaves had on blood sugar and investigated the effects on humans with Type 2 diabetes. Participants who received 1 g to 3 g of ground bay leaf per day for 30 days experienced a drop in blood glucose, cholesterol, and triglycerides. Because diabetes increases your risk of heart disease, the fact that bay leaves not only improved insulin function but simultaneously improved markers for heart disease is an encouraging result.

Another essential oil that doesn't get quite as much fanfare is Cypress (Cupressus sempervirens), which strengthens the vascular system and increases circulation while at the same time supports the detoxification of the lymphatic system. And, yet essential oil, Helichrysum (Helichrysum italicum) is a powerhouse all by itself as a natural anti-inflammatory; improving circulation and cleansing the blood. Both of these essential oils work well in a topical blend.

TIP: The U.S. Library of Medicine states evidence suggests that taking 1 gram ginger powder capsules three times daily (or 1-2 drops essential oil) for 45 days lowers triglyceride and cholesterol levels in people with high cholesterol.

Black Cumin (Nigella sativa) is another essential oil shown to lower plasma cholesterol and triglyceride levels due to its main constituent, thymoquinone.

There are many, many more essential oils to choose from.

Basil is used in relieving muscular aches and pains, colds and flu, hay fever, asthma, bronchitis, mental fatigue, anxiety, and depression. It is incredibly soothing and uplifting and is popular with massage therapists for alleviating tension and stress in their patients. When applied in dilution, Basil is reputed as being an excellent insect repellent while the linalool's mild analgesic properties are known to help in relieving insect bites and stings. It is also highly useful as an antispasmodic, as well as an antiemetic, antiseptic, carminative, cephalic, expectorant, and immune support. Basil essential oil works gradually, but effectively, in lowering bad cholesterol in the body. It is loaded with antioxidant, anti-inflammatory, and cholesterol-lowering actions. A recent study found that basil significantly reduced LDL ("bad") cholesterol when tested on rats with induced high cholesterol. At the same time, it increased the HDL ("good") cholesterol (Phytotherapy Research. 2006 Dec;20(12):1040-5.) This oil may irritate sensitive skin. Avoid use during pregnancy. Can be used topically, diffusion/inhalation, and internally. **Note:** Top

Bay Laurel (Laurus nobilis) includes chemical constituents Cineole and Linalool and has antiseptic, antibiotic, analgesic, anti-neuralgic, astringent, insecticidal and sedative properties. Bay is used in the treatment of rheumatism, muscular pain, circulation problems, colds, flu, dental infections and skin infections. Bay's high eugenol content may irritate the skin and mucous membranes, so dilution is necessary. Avoid use during pregnancy. Can be used topically, diffusion/inhalation, and internally. **Note:** Top

Bergamot (Citrus bergamia) is known as a powerful antidepressant by helping to release pent up emotions and accumulated stress. Bergamot is also known to be a powerful oil for raising HDL (good) cholesterol levels significantly, according to one study almost 65% and while lowering bad cholesterol with a significant decrease in triglycerides. This oil contains five different flavonoids that make it effective in lowering cholesterol, two of them have even been found to help prevent LDL (bad) cholesterol from depositing plaque. It is popular oil for controlling the appetite and aiding with weight loss. It also helps with controlling cholesterol levels since it contains large amounts of polyphenols which help to regulate metabolism and prevent cholesterol absorption. It is commonly used in many skin care creams and lotions because of its refreshing citrus nature. Bergamot is ideal for helping to calm inflamed skin and is an ingredient in some creams for eczema and psoriasis. Bergamot's chemical makeup has antiseptic properties, which help ward off infection and aid recovery. It is a favorite oil of aromatherapists in treating depression. Bergamot is also effective as an antispasmodic and helps to reduce leg cramps and is used for restless leg syndrome. It is also suitable for coughs and works as a digestive aid. The therapeutic properties of Bergamot include analgesic, antidepressant, antiseptic, antibiotic, antispasmodic, stomachic, calmative, cicatrizant, deodorant, digestive, febrifuge, vermifuge, and vulnerary. Bergamot essential oil has phototoxic properties and should not be used at more than 0.4% dilution on the skin, or if it is, the person should avoid exposure to the sun after use for 12-18 hours. It may also interfere with the activity of certain prescription drugs. Dr. Whitaker website suggested taking a dose of bergamot is 500–1,000 mg of a *standardized extract*, once or twice a day 20–30 minutes before meals. For maximum benefits, take bergamot twice a day for 60–90 days, reevaluate your lipid levels, and adjust your dose accordingly. Bergamot is safe and well tolerated. Can be used topically, diffusion/inhalation, and internally. **Note:** Top

Cassia (Cinnamomum Cassia) has antiseptic properties that are known to kill various types of bacteria and fungi. Cassia has been used as a tonic, carminative and stimulant for treating nausea, flatulence and diarrhea. Chinese and Japanese scientists have found that Cassia's sedative effect lowers high blood pressure. It helps maintain a healthy and functioning digestive system and improves blood circulation, reducing the risk of heart disease. Cassia's main chemical constituents are benzaldehyde, chavicol, cinnamic aldehyde, cinnamyl acetate, and linalool. Its antioxidant polyphenolic compounds are known to search for the formation of free radicals and prevent diseases such as cancer and diabetes. In the *Journal of Medicinal Food*, a 2005 study was published involving 15 diabetic men and women who were given either a cassia fiber supplement or placebo twice daily for two months. The results found that levels of serum triglycerides and low-density lipoprotein-cholesterol decreased in the cassia supplemented group. The therapeutic properties of Cassia are carminative, anti-diarrhea, antimicrobial and anti-emetic. It is a dermal irritant, dermal sensitizer and a mucous membrane irritant. Avoid use during pregnancy. Can be used topically (extremely diluted), diffusion/inhalation in a blend, and internally (diluted). **Note:** Middle

Cilantro or Coriander works as an analgesic, aphrodisiac, antispasmodic, carminative, deodorant, fungicidal and is revitalizing and stimulating. It relieves mental fatigue, migraine pain, stress and nervous debility. Coriander's warming effect is helpful for alleviating pain such as rheumatism, arthritis and muscle spasms. It contains antibacterial compounds preventing Salmonella, as well as possessing antimicrobial properties. The healing properties of Cilantro or Coriander oil are attributed to phytonutrient content, including carvone, geraniol, limonene, borneol, camphor, elemol, and linalool. Coriander's flavonoids include quercetin, kaempferol, rhamnetin, and epigenin, in addition to its active phenolic acid compounds, including caffeine and chlorogenic acid. Coriander has traditionally been referred to as an "anti-diabetic" herb and traditionally used in India for its anti-inflammatory properties. Recent studies conducted in the United States confirm Coriander's ability to reduce the amount of damaged fats (lipid peroxides) in cells, lower cholesterol levels of total and LDL, while increasing levels of HDL. Coriander oil is also beneficial for removing heavy metals and toxins from the body. Can be used topically, diffusion/inhalation, and internally. **Note:** Top

Cinnamon Bark (Cinnamomum zeylanicum) has a pleasant scent and is a perfect additive to creams, lotions, and soaps. It was traditionally used by the ancient Egyptians for foot massages and in love potions. Cinnamon has been used for rheumatism, kidney ailments, excess bile, to treat diarrhea, and other digestive problems. Cinnamon is known for lowering blood sugar and helps fight inflammation and infections in the body. Research studies show that taking ½ teaspoon of cinnamon powder per day will lower sugar levels and reduce cholesterol and triglycerides by up to 20%. The therapeutic properties of Cinnamon are analgesic, antiseptic, antibiotic, anti-diarrheal, antispasmodic, aphrodisiac, astringent, antiviral, cardiac, carminative, disinfectant, emmenagogue, insecticide, stimulant, stomachic, tonic and vermifuge. Cinnamon is known to elevate blood pressure. This oil may be irritating to the skin and mucous membranes – particularly in large doses. Sensitizing must be kept in mind when using Cinnamon in a blend for a friend or family member. This oil should always be used in dilution. Avoid use during pregnancy or if you have high blood pressure. Ceylon Cinnamon has ultra low (0.04%) coumarin levels compared to the common Cassia Cinnamon (4-8%). It can be taken in powder form according to the US Department of Health by mouth in amounts up to 1.2 teaspoon daily for six weeks, then rest. For oil, use 1-2 drops daily for five days, then rest on weekends. Can be used topically (extremely diluted), diffusion/inhalation in a blend, and internally (diluted). **Note:** Middle

Clary Sage (Salvia sclarea) can be used as a deodorant, antidepressant, and a sedative. Its analgesic and antispasmodic actions can decrease heart rate (Buckle, 1997) and is considered mildly hypotensive (Rovesti and Gattefosse, 1973). It is effective in combating oily hair and is a superior oil for acne, wrinkles and fine lines. Women experiencing hormonal changes and menopause symptoms such as hot flashes find this oil quite beneficial. Clary Sage's properties are antidepressant, anticonvulsive, antispasmodic, antiseptic, aphrodisiac, astringent, bactericidal, carminative, deodorant, digestive, emmenagogue, euphoric, hypotensive, nervine, sedative, stomachic, uterine and nerve tonic. Clary Sage Oil is non-toxic and non-sensitizing. Do not use during pregnancy or if you are at risk for breast cancer as it may have an estrogen-like effect on the body. Can be used topically, diffusion/inhalation, and internally. **Note:** Top-Middle

Clove Bud (Syzygium aromaticum) has a spicy rich scent and is useful for minor aches and pains, particularly dental pain because of its numerous effects on the oral tissues. An active ingredient in Clove is eugenol, which is an effective platelet inhibitor, that helps in preventing blood clot formation. Clove Bud can be used for acne, cuts and bruises, preventing infections and as a pain reliever. It helps with toothaches, mouth sores, rheumatism and arthritis. For the digestive system, it helps to prevent vomiting, diarrhea, flatulence, spasms and parasites, as well as bad breath. Clove oil is valuable for relieving respiratory problems, like bronchitis, asthma and tuberculosis. Its disinfecting feature makes it useful for infectious diseases. Clove oil's therapeutic properties are analgesic, antiseptic, antispasmodic, anti-neuralgic, carminative, anti-infectious, disinfectant, insecticide, tonic, stomachic, uterine, and stimulating. This oil may cause sensitization in some individuals and should be used in dilution. Avoid use during pregnancy. Can be used topically (extremely diluted), diffusion/inahalation in a blend, and internally (diluted). **Note:** Middle

Cypress (Cupressus sempervirens) assists with varicose veins and bodily fluids by improving circulation Cypress has strong antioxidant compounds and aids in removing toxins from the body acting such as Omega-3 oils. It is used to prevent excessive perspiration, particularly in the feet. It is good for hemorrhoids and oily skin, and acts as an astringent in skin care applications. It is extremely gentle and suitable for all skin types. This oil calms and soothes the nervous system. It is suitable for various female problems and is good for coughs and bronchitis.

Its properties include antibacterial, anti-infectious, anti-inflammatory, anti-rheumatic, antiseptic, antispasmodic, astringent, decongestant, diuretic, and vein tonic. Avoid use during pregnancy. Avoid long-term use with high-blood pressure. This oil is not intended for internal use (not GRAS) and is best used aromatically or topically. **Note:** Middle-Base

Dill is a stimulating, revitalizing, restoring, purifying, and a balancing oil. Its healing properties include antispasmodic, carminative, digestive, disinfectant, galactagogue, sedative, stomachic and sudorific. Dill is good for the digestive system and helps relieve cramps, diarrhea, flatulence, indigestion, and is known to whet the appetite. Studies on the effect of dill extract demonstrated positive activity on lipid profile, liver enzymes, gene expression and enzymatic activity in hamsters with high cholesterol. Dill Seed is non-toxic and non-irritating. Can be used topically, diffusion/inhalation, and internally. Avoid use during pregnancy. **Note:** Middle

Frankincense (Boswellia carterii) is highly prized in the aromatherapy industry. It contains monoterpenes that interfere with cholesterol synthesis and reduce cholesterol levels in the body. Frankincense is known to calm the mind and end mental chatter. It also helps to ease worry and agitation. The therapeutic properties of Frankincense oil are antiseptic, astringent, carminative, cicatrisant, cytophylactic, digestive, diuretic, emmenagogue, expectorant, sedative, tonic, uterine, and vulnerary. Frankincense is non-toxic, non-irritant and non-sensitizing. Can be used topically, diffusion/inhalation, and interanally. Avoid use during pregnancy. **Note:** Base

Garlic (Allium sativum) has antibacterial, antiseptic and antihypertensive properties that can be used to prevent infections as well as treat colds, bronchitis and flu symptoms. It is also a powerful detoxifier and rejuvenates the body. Garlic is recognized as a preventative of high blood pressure and heart disease when taken internally. It is extremely effective at reducing high cholesterol levels. Garlic's antiseptic, bactericidal and detoxifying properties make it a valuable essential oil in treating acne. Garlic has been used for thousands of years in preventing the infestation with intestinal worms, both in people and in animals, and is one of the best treatments for gastrointestinal infections. As an antibiotic, Garlic does not kill off the beneficial flora of the intestine as synthetic antibiotics do and is an effective treatment for cystitis. This oil must be properly diluted. Avoid use during pregnancy. Can be used internally (extremely diluted). **Note:** Top

Ginger (Zingiber officinale) contains curcumene that can help balance triglycerides. It is excellent for colds and flu, nausea (including motion sickness and morning sickness), rheumatism, coughs and circulation issues. Its warming properties help to relieve muscular cramps, spasms, aches and eases stiffness in joints. Ginger contains antioxidant compounds that can assist the body with waste elimination and help reduce inflammation which in turn promotes healthy circulation. It is a natural anti-depressant along with anti-hemorrhagic properties which are considered to be beneficial for the heart. The essential oil also facilitates the breakdown of sugar and its absorption. Ginger's healing properties include analgesic, anti-inflammatory, antiseptic, antispasmodic, carminative, tonic, diaphoretic, expectorant, and antiemetic. It may irritate sensitive skin. Can be used topically, diffusion/inahalation, and internally. **Note**: Base

Goldenrod (Solidago virgaurea) is known to support the circulatory system, urinary tract, and liver function. It has relaxing and calming effects with anti-inflammatory, antihypertensive, diuretic, and liver tonic properties. Goldenrod is helpful for the cardiovascular system, bladder infection, congestive cough, diphtheria, diuretic, dyspepsia, fibrillation, heart tonic (stimulant), hypertension, hepatitis, impotence, influenza, fatty liver, liver congestion, nervousness, neuropathy, respiratory mucus, sleep disorders, tachycardia, tonsillitis, and pharyngitis. Goldenrod could possibly cause skin sensitivity. Avoid use during pregnancy. This oil is not GRAS and should be used topically and inhalation only. **Note:** Middle

Grapefruit (Citrus × paradisi) eases muscle fatigue and stiffness, relieves nervous exhaustion and alleviates depression. This potent essential oil helps to reduce cholesterol levels by detoxifying the blood acting as a cholesterol reducing agent. Grapefruit essential oil is a favorite oil for weight loss due to its chemical component d-limonene that aids in the release of fatty acids in the blood. It is known to reduce lipid peroxidation and cholesterol levels. Grapefruit helps to clear congested, oily and acne prone skin. Grapefruit is sometimes added to creams and lotions as a natural toner and cellulite treatment. Grapefruit's therapeutic properties are antiviral, astringent, antidepressant, antiseptic, decongestant, diuretic, and tonic. It can cause photosensitivity. Can be used topically (diluted), diffusion/inhalation, and internally. **Note**: Top

---

SPECIAL NOTE: There is often confusion regarding whether it is safe to use grapefruit essential oil with certain medications. Grapefruit essential oil is cold-pressed from the rind. Any concerns with medication comes from the juice of the fruit. Therefore, it is completely safe

Helichrysum (Helichrysum italicum) is an effective oil for the chelation of plaque in blood vessels. It is also good for acne, bruises, boils, burns, cuts, dermatitis, eczema, irritated skin and wounds. It supports the body through post-viral fatigue and convalescence, and can also be used to repair skin damaged by psoriasis, eczema or ulceration. Helichrysum's therapeutic properties include anti-inflammatory, antibacterial, analgesic, antiseptic, antispasmodic, antifungal, antiviral, antimicrobial, and as a tonic for the nervous system. This oil is non-toxic, non-irritating and non-sensitizing. Please check with your healthcare provider before use during pregnancy. This oil is GRAS and can be used topically, by inhalation, and internally. **Note:** Base

Lavender (Lavandula angustifolia) is most commonly used for burns and the healing of skin. It is also known to help regulate and maintain cholesterol levels. It has been demonstrated that inhalation of lavender essential oil (0.1-0.2mg/m^3 of air) can reduce the cholesterol content in the aorta and atherosclerotic plaques, but without affecting blood cholesterol (Nikolaevskii et al. 1990, cited by Shaaban, El-ghorab and Shibamato 2012). With its calming and sedative qualities, it can help relax the mind and body and dilate the blood vessels for proper blood flow. It has antiseptic and analgesic properties that eases the pain of a burn and prevents infection. Lavender also has cytophylactic properties that promote rapid healing and reduce scarring. Lavender does an excellent job at balancing oil production in the skin as well as clearing blemishes and evening skin tone, and even helps to hydrate dry skin. Lavender is indicated for all skin types and can be used at any step in your skin care regimen. Lavender is beneficial for colds, flu, asthma, high blood pressure, and migraines. It is also excellent for helping with insomnia. The therapeutic properties of Lavender oil are antiseptic, analgesic, anticonvulsant, antidepressant, antirheumatic, antispasmodic, anti-inflammatory, antiviral, bactericide, carminative, cholagogue, cicatrisant, cordial, cytophylactic, decongestant, deodorant, diuretic, emmenagogue, hypotensive, nervine, rubefacient, sedative, sudorific and vulnerary. Lavender is non-toxic, non-irritating and non-sensitizing. Do not use during the first trimester of pregnancy. Can be used topcally, diffusion/inhalation, and internally. **Note:** Middle

Lemon (Citrus Limon) is recognized as a cleanser and antiseptic with refreshing and cooling properties. For the skin and hair, Lemon is used for its cleansing effect, as well as for treating cuts and boils. This oil's fresh scent is treasured for improving concentration, reducing acidity in the body while assisting with digestion and eliminating cellulite, rheumatism, arthritis, and gout. It is beneficial for the circulatory system and aids with blood flow, reduces blood pressure and helps with nosebleeds. Lemon oil can be used to help reduce a fever, relieve throat infections and bronchitis, and heal cold sores, herpes, and insect bites. Lemon's therapeutic properties are anti-anemic, antimicrobial, antirheumatic, anti-sclerotic, antiseptic, bactericidal, carminative, cicatrisant, depurative, diaphoretic, diuretic, febrifuge, haemostatic, hypotensive, insecticidal, rubefacient, tonic and vermifuge. Lemon is non-toxic but may cause skin irritation for some. It is also phototoxic and should be avoided prior to exposure to direct sunlight. Can be used topically (diluted), diffusion/inhalation and internally. **Note:** Top

Lemongrass is known for its invigorating qualities and makes an excellent antidepressant. This essential oil is known to promote blood circulation and lower cholesterol levels by dilating the blood vessels, allowing uninterrupted blood flow. Lemongrass contains compounds called terpenoids that inhibit the production of mevalonic acid, which helps produce cholesterol. It also helps reduce inflammation, which can contribute to plaque build-up. It has been reported that these compounds inhibit the production of mevalonic acid, an intermediary in the production of cholesterol and the target of many cholesterol-lowering pharmaceutical drugs. It has potent analgesic and anti-inflammatory properties. Lemongrass not only tones but fortifies the nervous system and can be used in the bath for soothing muscular nerves and pain with its potent analgesic and anti-inflammatory qualities. Lemongrass has an outstanding reputation for keeping insects away, controlling perspiration and for treating athletics' foot. This oil relieves the symptoms of jet lag, helps with nervousness and anxiety, and clears headaches. It is useful for respiratory conditions such as sore throats, laryngitis and fever and helps prevent spreading of infectious diseases when diffused. It is also good for colitis, indigestion and gastroenteritis. The therapeutic properties of Lemongrass oil are analgesic, antidepressant, antimicrobial, antipyretic, antiseptic, astringent, bactericidal, carminative, deodorant, diuretic, febrifuge, fungicidal, galactagogue, insecticidal, nervine, nervous system sedative and tonic. Avoid use with individuals with glaucoma. Use caution in prostatic hyperplasia and with skin hypersensitivity or damaged skin. Avoid use during the first trimester of pregnancy. Avoid if you have a history of high blood pressure. Safe for topical and ingestion if diluted properly. A suggested safe limit for humans (based on an experiment in rats) is 0.7 mg/kg/day of the essential oil. Can be used topically, diffusion/inhalation, and internally. **Note:** Top

Lime (Citrus × aurantiifolia) has a crisp, refreshing citrus scent with uplifting and revitalizing properties that help with depression. It acts as an astringent on the skin and helps clear oily skin. Lime cools fevers due to colds and flu, eases coughs and strengthens the immune system as well as treats bronchitis, asthma, and sinusitis. Lime oil is also helpful for arthritis, rheumatism, poor circulation, and in eliminating cellulite and obesity. The therapeutic properties of Lime are antiseptic, antiviral, astringent, aperitif, bactericidal, disinfectant, febrifuge, haemostatic, restorative and tonic. Lime is considered phototoxic; users should avoid direct sunlight after application. Can be used topically, diffusion/inhalation, and internally. **Note**: Top

Marjoram (Origanum marjorana) is known for helping combat stress and anxiety. Marjoram's chemical constituents of aldehydes, in the form of citral and geranyl acetate, aid in lowering the blood pressure, dilating vessels (Tiran, 1996). It is a comforting oil that can be massaged into the abdomen during menstruation, or added to a warm compress to ease discomfort. It is useful for treating tired aching muscles or in a sports massage. Marjoram's pain relieving properties are useful for rheumatic pains, sprains, and spasms, as well as swollen joints and achy muscles. It can be added to a warm or hot bath at the first sign of a cold. This oil is helpful for asthma and other respiratory complaints and has a calming effect on emotions, especially for hyperactive people. It soothes the digestive system and helps with indigestion, constipation and flatulence. Marjoram is superb as a relaxant and is useful for headaches, migraines and insomnia. Marjoram is relaxing and quiets the mind and obsessive over-thinking. Marjoram's therapeutic properties are analgesic, antispasmodic, anaphrodisiac, antiseptic, antiviral, bactericidal, carminative, cephalic, cordial, diaphoretic, digestive, diuretic, emmenagogue, expectorant, fungicidal, hypotensive, laxative, nervine, sedative, stomachic, vasodilator and vulnerary. It can also be used in masculine, oriental, and herbal-spicy perfumes and colognes. Marjoram is generally non-toxic, non-irritating and non-sensitizing. Use with caution if you have low blood pressure. Avoid use during pregnancy. Can be used topically, diffusion/inhalation, and internally. **Note**: Middle

Myrrh (Commiphora myrrh) is characterized as antimicrobial, antifungal, astringent, healing, tonic, stimulant, carminative, expectorant, diaphoretic, locally antiseptic, immune stimulant, bitter, circulatory stimulant, anti-inflammatory, and antispasmodic. As an anti-inflammatory, it has been reported to lower cholesterol levels and blood pressure in the body. This oil is well known for its spiritual aspects, but is also suitable for treating female complaints, skin ailments, as well as detoxifying the body and expelling mucus and phlegm from the lungs and helps with ailments such as colds, coughs, sore throats and bronchitis. Myrrh is used for diarrhea, dyspepsia, flatulence and hemorrhoids. It is commonly used for the treatment of mouth and gum infections, ulcers, gingivitis, and pyorrhea. Myrrh is also good for skin infections such as boils, skin ulcers, bedsores, ringworm, wounds that won't heal, eczema and athletics' foot. Myrrh can be possibly toxic in high concentrations. Can be used topically, diffusion/inhalation, and internally. **Note:** Base

Melissa (Melissa officinalis) also commonly called Lemon Balm, is well known for its antidepressant and uplifting properties. Its healing properties include antidepressant, anti-inflammatory, antiviral, antispasmodic, bactericidal, carminative, cordial, diaphoretic, emmenagogue, nervine, sedative, stomachic, sudorific, and tonic. Melissa has strong sedative qualities and treats emotional trauma and shock. It is considered non-sensitizing and non-toxic. Lemon balm has shown antioxidant activity in several studies (Apak et al 2006, Canadanovic-Brunet et al 2008, Ferreira et al 2006, Hohmann et al 1999, Lopez et al 2007). An extract of lemon balm reduced blood cholesterol and lipid levels in rats fed a high fat and alcohol diet (Bolkent et al 2005). Interestingly, the extract also increased glutathione levels and reduced lipid peroxidation in the liver, demonstrating a hepatoprotective effect. Please check with your healthcare provider before use during pregnancy. Can be used topically, diffusion/inhalation, and internally. **Note:** Middle-Top

Neroli (Citrus aurantium) increases circulation and stimulates new cell growth. It prevents scarring and stretch marks, and is useful in treating skin conditions linked to emotional stress. Any type of skin can benefit from this oil, although it is particularly nourishing for dry, irritated or sensitive skin. Neroli regulates oiliness, minimizes enlarged pores, and helps clear acne and blemished skin, especially if the skin lacks moisture. With regular treatment, it can reduce the appearance of fragile or broken capillaries and varicose veins. Neroli is useful for dry, sensitive and mature skin as it helps improves elasticity. It is also known to help relieve muscle spasms and heart palpitations. It provides comfort and strength emotionally and helps to release repressed emotions. Neroli's therapeutic properties are antidepressant, antiseptic, anti-infectious, antispasmodic, aphrodisiac, bactericidal, carminative, cicatrisant, cytophylactic, cordial, deodorant, digestive, sedative and tonic. This oil is non-toxic and non-sensitizing. Avoid use during pregnancy. Use topically or by inhalation. Oral ingestion is not recommended unless under the supervision of a qualified health practitioner. This oil is not GRAS and should be used topically (extremely diluted) and through inhalation only. **Note:** Middle-Top

Orange, Sweet (Citrus sinensis) works as an antidepressant, antiseptic, antispasmodic, aphrodisiac, carminative, deodorant, stimulant (nervous) and tonic for the cardiac and circulatory system. It helps with dull skin, the flu, gums, and stress. This oil is truly uplifting, excellent for stress while calming digestive problems and eliminating toxins. It stimulates the lymphatic system and supports the formation of collagen in the skin. Orange Essential Oil contains 85-95% limonene and is the highest level of d-limonene next to grapefruit oil. It is considered phototoxic; therefore exposure to sunlight should be avoided. Can be used topically, diffusion/inhalation, and internally. **Note:** Top

Oregano (Origanum vulgare) is considered nature's cure-all due to its high carvacrol and thymol content. This oil's potent properties include antiviral, antifungal, antibacterial and antiparasitic. In topical applications, oregano can be used to treat skin infections, cuts and wounds. Oregano's anti-inflammatory properties make it effective against swelling and pain caused by rheumatism. Due to its nutrient content including omega-3, fiber and the semi-essential amino acid arginine, oregano is a true support to the heart. Research has shown that consuming the antioxidant vitamins and minerals in oregano can help reduce cholesterol levels and triglyceride levels ("Hypotensive effects of carvacrol on the blood pressure of normotensive rats." Planta Med 13:73;1365-71). In addition, oregano oil helps normalize blood pressure levels, while its antibacterial properties help prevent infection-related heart disease. Oregano oil is known as a natural cholesterol-reducing agent. However, caution needs to be exercised when using it as it may interact with medications such as blood thinners. Oregano is both a dermal irritant and a mucous membrane irritant. Avoid use during pregnancy. Can be used topically (extremely diluted), diffusion/inhalation in a blend, and internally (diluted). **Note:** Top

Peppermint (Mentha × piperita) has long been credited as being useful in combating stomach ailments, soothing to the digestive system. Great for headaches, travel sickness and jet lag. It is viewed as an antispasmodic and antimicrobial agent. Most people know it as a flavoring or scenting agent in food, beverages, skin and hair care products (where it has a cooling effect by constricting capillaries and helps with bruises and sore joints). Its properties include antifungal, antiseptic, antispasmodic, astringent, anti-inflammatory, analgesic, carminative, febrifuge, decongestant, expectorant, and stimulating to the circulatory and immune system. Peppermint can be sensitizing due to the menthol content. Do not use if you have cardiac fibrillation. Please check with your healthcare provider regarding use during pregnancy. Avoid if you have a history of high blood pressure. Maximum oral daily dose is 152mg and maximum dermal dose is 5.4%. Can be used topically, diffusion/inhalation, and internally. **Note**: Top-Middle

Petitgrain (Citrus aurantium) is believed to have uplifting properties and is used for calming anger and stress. It is commonly used in the skin care industry for acne, oily skin, and as a deodorizing agent. Petitgrain is valued for its ability to reduce pain and spasms in the lower intestines. Its calming qualities make it a favorite for insomnia. This oil's properties include antidepressant, antiseptic, antispasmodic, deodorant, immuno-support and stimulant, tonic and sedative for the nervous system. Petitgrain is generally considered non-toxic, non-irritant, and non-sensitizing. Can be used topically, diffusion/inhalation, and internally. **Note:** Top

Roman Chamomile (Anthemis nobilis) helps relieve nervous stress of any kind, while easing frustration, resentment and depression. It is good for most skin types, acne, allergies, boils, burns, eczema, inflamed skin conditions, wounds, menstrual pain, premenstrual syndrome, headache, insomnia, restless leg syndrome, and nervous tension. The therapeutic properties of Roman Chamomile oil are analgesic, antispasmodic, antiseptic, antibiotic, anti-inflammatory, anti-infectious, antidepressant, antineuralgic, antiphlogistic, antiseptic, antispasmodic, bactericidal, carminative, cholagogues, cicatrisant, emmenagogue, febrifuge, hepatic, sedative, nervine, digestive, tonic, sudorific, stomachic, vermifuge and vulnerary. It is non-toxic and non-irritant. A 2006 review of clinical trials reported a number of beneficial effects in vitro and animal tests, suggests cholesterol-lowering effects for Chamomile. It also has blood and liver cleansing detoxifying properties. Chamomile contains coumarin, so care should be taken to avoid potential drug interactions with blood thinners. This oil should not be used by anyone who is allergic to ragweed. Avoid use during the first and second trimester of pregnancy. Can be used topically, diffusion/inhalation, and internally. **Note:** Middle

Rosemary (Rosmarinus officinalis) improves circulation, helping to relieve aches and pains and arthritis, with its analgesic properties. It can also help reduce cholesterol levels in the body due to its chemical component, camphene. Rosemary contains a very high level of antioxidants which helps with cholesterol. Rosemary stimulates cell renewal and improves dry or mature skin, eases lines and wrinkles, and heals burns and wounds. It can clear acne, blemishes or dull dry skin by fighting bacteria and regulating oil secretions. This warming oil improves circulation and can reduce the appearance of broken capillaries and varicose veins. It tones and tightens the skin and is helpful for sagging skin. Rosemary helps to overcome mental fatigue and sluggishness by stimulating and strengthening the entire nervous system. It also enhances mental clarity while aiding alertness and concentration. It is also beneficial to use in stressful conditions. Rosemary is generally non-toxic and non-sensitizing but is not suitable for people with epilepsy. Rosemary's therapeutic properties are analgesic, anti-inflammatory, anti-rheumatic, antiseptic, astringent, antispasmodic, antiviral, decongestant, diuretic, expectorant, restorative, and stimulant. Avoid use during pregnancy. Can be used topically, diffusion/inhalation, and internally. **Note**: Middle

Sage (Salvia officinalis) is believed to calm the nerves, assist with grief and depression, and with female sterility as well as menopausal problems. For topical applications, Sage is reputed to relieve swelling, and relieve pain caused by rheumatism. It may be used to reduce pore size, heal wounds and infections, and assist with skin conditions such as psoriasis and dermatitis. The therapeutic properties of Sage oil are anti-inflammatory, antibacterial, antiseptic, antispasmodic, astringent, digestive, diuretic, emmenagogue, febrifuge, hypertensive, laxative, stomachic and tonic. This oil should not be used during pregnancy or by persons suffering from epilepsy. Use in low concentration. Can be used topically (extremely diluted), diffusion/inhalation, and internally. **Note:** Top-Middle

Tangerine (Citrus reticulate) is a refreshing and rejuvenating oil. Its aroma clears the mind and can help to eliminate emotional confusion. Tangerine is truly comforting, soothing and warming oil used in perfumes and soaps. This oil is good for weeping wounds and cuts that won't heal. Its healing properties include antispasmodic, carminative, digestive stimulant, diuretic, sedative, stimulant for the lymphatic system, and tonic agent. As a powerful depurative, it helps to remove toxic and unwanted substances like uric acid and excess salt from the body via sweat and urine. It contains 85-98.6% limonene. Like other citrus oils, tangerine oil can be phototoxic. Skin should not be exposed to sunlight after topical use. Similarly, the oil should be diluted well before use on the skin. Can be used topically, diffusion/inhalation, and internally. **Note:** Top

Turmeric (Curcuma longa) is viewed as a strong relaxant and balancer. It has historical applications as an antiseptic aid for skin care used in treating acne and facial hair in women. It is an analgesic for painful joint conditions such as rheumatism. This oil makes a wonderful digestive aid and helps to reduce excess fluid. Its therapeutic properties include analgesic, anti-inflammatory, carminative, tonic, and diuretic. One of its principle compounds, Curcumin, a polyphenolic compound is what gives it a deep orange color. In vitro and laboratory animal studies found that the curcumin has anti-tumor, antioxidant, antiarthritic, anti-amyloid, anti-ischemic, and anti-inflammatory properties. This popular herb is rich in antioxidants which helps to control blood LDL ("bad") cholesterol levels. Turmeric contains lots of minerals like calcium, iron, potassium, manganese, copper, zinc, and magnesium. Potassium plays a very important part in cell and body fluids which helps control heart rate and blood pressure. Turmeric essential oil has potential irritating and toxic effects when used in large concentrations. Avoid use during pregnancy. Can be used topically, diffusion/inhalation, and internally. Only use GRAS very high-quality oil for internal use. **Note:** Base

Ylang Ylang (Cananga odorata) assists with problems such as high blood pressure due to its content of alcohols and cadinene, which is hypotensive (Tiran 1996), rapid breathing and heartbeat, nervous conditions, as well as impotence and frigidity. Ylang Ylang is renowned as a treatment for arterial hypertension and tachycardia (Rose, 1994). According to a 2005 study, which compared the free radical scavenging properties, it was the most effective remedy tested. This oil is best suited for use in the perfumery and skin care industries due to it having a balancing effect on sebum and is useful for both oily and dry skin types. The therapeutic properties of Ylang Ylang are antidepressant, antiseborrheic, antiseptic, aphrodisiac, hypotensive, nervine and sedative. Ylang Ylang may cause sensitivity in some people and excessive use of it may lead to headaches and nausea. This oil is not recommended if you have low blood pressure. Can be used topically, diffusion/inhalation, and internally. **Note:** Base

HOW ESSENTIAL OILS HELP LOWER CHOLESTEROL

Incorporating essential oils and natural remedies such as aromatherapy and relaxation techniques into your life can be very beneficial for a number of health conditions. Most essential oils are safe and free of adverse side effects when used properly. However, as with any substance you are introducing into your body, it is important to use them intelligently.

While many people with high cholesterol can benefit from certain essential oils that contain terpenoid compounds such as geraniol and citral that decrease cholesterol levels, there are some factors you must consider:

Dosage – Dose is the most significant factor in essential oil usage. Some essential oils used in the wrong doses such as in too high of a concentration have been found (in animal and laboratory studies) to cause adverse effects in the body. Some essential oils can damage the skin, liver and other organs if misused.

Quality – The purity of the essential oil is important. Even when an oil is labeled as pure, it may be adulterated with added synthetic chemicals or other, similar smelling, cheaper essential oils or with a vegetable oil. Make sure your oils are therapeutic quality.

Application – An essential oil that is safe when applied in one way may not be safe when used in another way. Some oils are considered safe if inhaled, and yet may be irritating if applied to the skin in concentration. For instance, citrus oils such as Bergamot and Lemon can cause phototoxicity (severe burn to the skin) if a person is exposed to the sun after topical application. However, this would not result from inhalation.

Lifestyle – Since untreated high cholesterol can lead to more serious health issues such as heart disease, it is important to combine your use of essential oils with diet and lifestyle changes to achieve success with your natural remedy.

Drug Interaction – If you're currently under a doctor's care for high cholesterol, talk to your doctor before starting any treatment program with essential oils. You will want to make sure that your use of oils will not interfere with medications you are prescribed.

Another option is to find a naturopath to talk about holistic health care that looks at your health as a whole, instead of treating symptoms of individual conditions. As you study and research therapeutic quality essential oils, you will find these are a great way to complement your whole body care, instead of taking a handful of pills every day for multiple medical issues.

To monitor your progress, have your cholesterol levels checked after two to three months.

SPECIAL NOTE: Essential oils are not a "magic bullet." The suggestions of use for essential oils in this book are for you to use as complementary care to the healthcare plan you already have in place. It may be necessary for you to make changes in a proper diet and other lifestyle modifications for all things to work together. High Cholesterol is a grave health concern and should be treated properly. If you do not achieve satisfactory results in normalizing your cholesterol, please seek professional medical help.

SMART TIP: For best results in lowering your cholesterol, only purchase oils that are available in capsule form and labeled as "standardized extracts." When a package is labeled as standardized extracts, this means that they are diluted and safe for consumption. Follow the dosage instructions listed on the manufacturer's label.

CAN ESSENTIAL OILS BE INGESTED?

The concept of ingesting essential oils is nothing new – evidence has shown that this was common practice throughout ancient civilizations. However, most of us already ingest essential oils every day without realizing, as they are commonly used to add flavoring in the confectionery industry. Hundreds of everyday products, such as toothpaste and cola, rely on essential oils for their unique flavor. This only serves to prove that ingesting essential oils is not toxic per se – when used with due care, they can be a wonderful addition to our daily diet. Some experts believe the ingestion of essential oils is not only harmless but can be positively beneficial to our internal health and well-being.

Yes, essential oils do contain some toxic components, but when using minuscule amounts, they are rendered harmless. Nutmeg is known to produce psychotropic and hallucinogenic effects, with the potential to cause acute poisoning if eaten whole. However, the average person would have to consume at least 100ml of nutmeg essential oil to reach a lethal dose – far more than would ever be required use for a blend.

HOW ESSENTIAL OILS ARE METABOLIZED BY THE BODY

While ingesting essential oils through the oral route, care should be taken due to the potential toxicity of some essential oils. Essential oil compounds and their metabolites that are ingested are absorbed in the digestive tract and enter the blood stream where they are distributed to their target organs.

Various research findings confirm that essential oils are rapidly absorbed into the blood stream after administration through dermal, oral, or pulmonary (via inhalation) route. They then cross the blood-brain barrier and attach to the various receptors present in the central nervous system and produce their effects of improving sleep, relaxing the mind and body, benefiting digestion, and more.

It has also been confirmed in studies that the majority of the components in essential oils metabolized in the body are either eliminated or excreted by the kidneys, or exhaled by the lungs in the form of carbon dioxide. Various research findings confirm that essential oils are rapidly absorbed into the blood stream after administration through dermal, oral, or pulmonary (via inhalation) route.

TOXICITY OF ESSENTIAL OILS

Certain essential oils could have irritation potential and can be toxic if large doses are ingested. For this reason, only a drop or two is used.

Some of the short-term complications of ingesting essential oils in large doses are:

- Essential oils may cause burning of the mucous membranes of the oral cavity, throat, and esophagus when not properly diluted.
- Essential oils may lead to occurrence of reflux by irritating the digestive tract if taken undiluted.
- Certain essential oils may cause symptoms of nausea, vomiting and/or diarrhea.
- Some essential oils may also interfere with certain medications and can make them useless or lead to complications such as seizures.
- Essential oils have the potential to interfere with anesthesia.

- Essential oils can elevate the liver enzymes.

Some of the long-term complications of ingesting essential oils are:

- Ingesting essential oils long term can cause liver cancer, liver failure, enlargement of liver, and fatty liver disease (all of these complications occur due to undue stress on the liver by metabolizing the essential oils)
- Kidney failure.

TIP: Daniel Pénoël, M.D. recommends using essential oils in food preparation as they purify the body, enhance the immune system and generate endorphins.

HOW ARE ESSENTIAL OILS EXCRETED FROM THE BODY?

When essential oils are applied topically or inhaled, they initially bypass the liver and interact with the target organs to produce their desired effect. Finally, the essential oils metabolites enter the blood and lymph, are redirected to the liver and ultimately excreted via the intestinal and urinary tract.

In the case of oral ingestion of essential oils, they are absorbed into the blood stream and directed to the liver by the time they have reached the small intestine. In the liver, the essential oil molecules are metabolized to form various phytochemicals which are further broken down. The essential oil can become toxic when the liver prefers to metabolize other substances first, instead of the essential oil phytochemicals. This can lead to accumulation of the phytochemicals in the liver. These phytochemicals can sometimes reach toxic amounts. For instance, a common bioactive fraction of peppermint oil, 1,8 cineole, is not preferred by the liver and it can quickly accumulate to dangerous levels causing liver failure.

Essential oils are not water-soluble but are made water-soluble by various enzymes found in the liver. From there, they are excreted by the kidneys via urine. When an essential oil component is introduced to the body at a faster rate than the liver can convert it into a water-soluble form, liver toxicity can result. (This can happen from any mode of entry, not just ingestion.)

Different protocols exist for ingesting essential oils orally. This largely depends on the body part to which the action of essential oil is targeted. You should be aware of these protocols before ingesting essential oils orally.

Be sure to exercise caution if you are taking any medications, as their interaction with essential oil components may hinder their effectiveness. If in doubt, consult a qualified Aromatherapist for advice.

Essential oils can be quite useful if proper protocol is followed when you are ingesting them orally. Take care to be aware of the dosage, the effects and potential toxicity of the particular essential oil you are planning to ingest orally. If taken in small doses (preferably a couple of drops initially), essential oils can be used effectively to relieve many physical and emotional health issues.

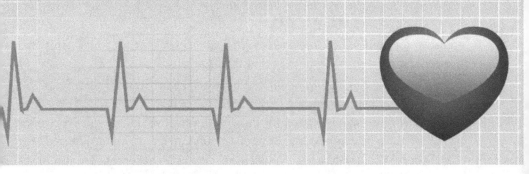

ESSENTIAL OIL SAFETY

In general, essential oils are safe to use for aromatherapy and therapeutic purposes. Nevertheless, safety must be exercised due to their potency and high concentration. Please read and follow these guidelines to obtain the maximum effectiveness and benefits.

- Avoid sunbathing, tanning booths, or saunas immediately after using essential oils.
- Be careful to avoid getting essential oils in the eyes. If you do splash a drop or two of essential oil in the eyes, use a small amount of olive oil (or another carrier oil) to dilute the essential oil and absorb with a washcloth. If severe, seek medical attention immediately.
- Take extra precaution when using oils with children. Never use undiluted essential oils on babies and always store your essential oils out of the reach of children.
- Never take essential oils internally without knowledge of its effect or proper usage. Seek the advice of a knowledgeable medical practitioner or another qualified clinical aromatherapist.
- If a dangerous quantity of essential oil has been ingested, immediately drink olive oil and induce vomiting. The olive oil will help in slowing down its

absorption and will dilute the essential oil. Do not drink water—this will speed up the absorption of the essential oil.

- Most essential oils should be diluted before applying topically. Pay attention to safety guidelines—certain essential oils, such as Cinnamon and Clove Bud, may cause skin irritation for those with sensitive skin. If you experience slight redness or itchiness, put olive oil (or any carrier oil) on the affected area and cover with a soft cloth. The olive oil acts as an absorbent fat and binds to the oil diluting its strength and allowing it to be immediately removed. Aloe Vera gel also works well as an alternative to olive oil. Never use water to dilute essential oil—this will cause it to spread and enlarge the affected area. Redness or irritation may last 20 minutes to an hour.

- Never use oils undiluted on your skin. Always dilute with a carrier oil. If redness, burning, itching, or irritation occurs, stop using oil immediately. Be sure to wash hands after handling pure, undiluted essential oils.

- For sensitive skin or when using a new oil, perform a "Skin Patch Test." If irritation occurs, discontinue use of such oil or blend. See section, Skin Patch Test.

- If you are pregnant, lactating, suffer from epilepsy, have cancer, liver damage, or another medical condition, use essential oils under the care and supervision of a qualified Aromatherapist or medical practitioner.

- If taking prescription drugs, check for interaction between medicine and essential oils (if any) to avoid interference with certain prescription medications.

- To prevent contact sensitization (redness or irritation of skin due to repeated use of same individual oil) use different oils.

- Rotating essential oils is the most efficient and safest way to use them. Choose one essential oil and try it first for a couple of weeks, then switch to another oil.

- Be sure to check with your doctor before using essential oils. Some prescription medications contraindicate the use of some essential oils.

- Less is best when taking essential oils internally. Take fewer drops at one time every 4-6 hours, versus more at one time.

- After two to three months, have your cholesterol checked to monitor your progress.

SKIN PATCH TEST

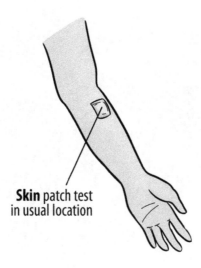

Skin patch test
in usual location

Certain essential oils can cause sensitization or an allergic reaction in some individuals. When using a new oil for the first time, you may want to perform a simple skin patch test on the inside of your arm or your chest. Place one drop of the essential oil into a carrier oil. Apply one drop on the skin and cover with a bandage. If skin becomes irritated and red, remove the bandage and immediately wash the area with soap and water. If after 12 hours no irritation has occurred, it is safe to use on the skin.

For someone who tends to be highly allergic, here is a simple test to determine if he or she is sensitive to a particular carrier oil and essential oil.

1. First, rub a drop of carrier oil onto the upper chest. In 12 hours, check for redness or other skin irritation.
2. If the skin remains clear, place 1 drop of selected essential oil in 15 drops of the same carrier oil, and again rub into the upper chest. If no skin reaction appears after 12 hours, it is safe to use the carriers and the essential oil.

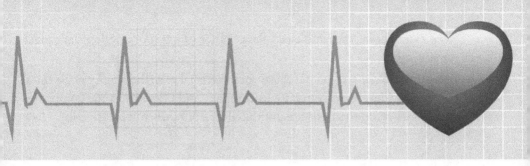

ESSENTIAL OILS
STORAGE AND SAFETY

Because essential oils contain no fatty acids, they are not susceptible to rancidity like vegetable oils – but you will want to protect them from the degenerative effects of heat, light, and air. Store them in tightly sealed, dark glass bottles away from any heat source. Properly stored oils can maintain their quality for years. (Citrus oils are less stable and should not be stored longer than six months after opening.)

ESSENTIAL OIL STORAGE TIPS:

- Keep oils tightly closed and out of reach of children.
- Always read and follow all labeled warnings and cautions.
- Do not purchase essential oils with rubber glass dropper tops. Essential oils are highly concentrated and will turn the rubber to a gum, thus ruining the oil.
- Make a note of when the bottle of essential oil was opened and its shelf life.
- Many essential oils will remove furniture finish. Use care when handling open bottles.

- Keep essential oil vials and clear glass bottles in a box or another dark place for storing.
- Be selective of where you purchase your essential oils. The quality of essential oil varies widely from company to company. Additionally, some companies may falsely claim their oils are undiluted and pure when they are not.

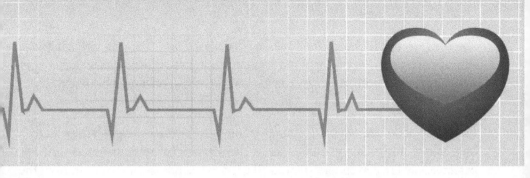

HOW TO USE ESSENTIAL OILS FOR CHOLESTEROL

There are several options available for lowering your cholesterol levels in both allopathic and alternative medicine. Many people today are able to regulate their cholesterol levels with the help of therapeutic quality essential oils along with vigilance and commitment to a healthy diet and lifestyle.

Various mechanisms can be used to deliver essential oils to target sites in the body. Common routes of administration include topically, inhalation, and ingestion. Essential oils may also be given by rectal suppositories. Regardless of which route of administration is used, the essential oils have to travel to the site of action with either the help of blood, nerves or oxygen (when inhalation route is used).

Using a combination of these three approaches for reducing your cholesterol will ensure success.

Topically seems to be one of the most easiest ways. For example, massage stimulates circulation of the blood while reducing muscular tension, aches, and pain. In addition, it significantly reduces stress and can offer comfort and peace of mind, allowing healing to take place.

Inhalation of certain essential oil's vapors, on the other hand, triggers the olfactory bulb which immediately sends a neurochemical signal to neuro-receptors. For example, smelling lavender essential oil triggers the release of serotonin from the raphe nucleus in the brain and produces a calmative effect.

Ingestion of certain essential oils may serve to be the most efficient method for absorption into the bloodstream for promoting healthy cholesterol levels. They are absorbed into systemic circulation via the digestive tract. However, when taken orally, essential oils may lose some of the active principal compounds due to the first pass hepatic metabolism. There are several methods for taking essential oils. In this study, internal use will comprise of consuming essential oils by mouth in a vegetable capsule, or by adding oil to honey, or on a sugar cube. Essential oils taken by mouth not in a capsule may be absorbed through the cheeks, the tongue or the lining of the throat.

Essential oils are highly concentrated and potent – treat like you would with any other highly concentrated pharmaceutical. It is recommended when using essential oils internally to seek the advice of a certified medical practitioner who is also trained in aromatherapy or a certified aromatherapist who is also trained in internal ingestion for the best protocol.

INHALATION

Essential oils can easily be absorbed via inhalation and enter the bloodstream to deliver healing constituents throughout the body. Inhalation presents the least amount of risk with most individuals.

- **Diffuse** – Use a nebulizer to diffuse your choice of oils for ½ hour, three times a day. You may want to use one specific essential oil (with no carrier oil added). Or, you may blend a combination of essential oils together.
- **Cup Hands** – Place 2-3 drops of your chosen essential oil in your hand and rub your palms together. Cup hands over your nose and inhale deeply.
- **Inhaler** – Add 1-2 drops of essential oil to a tissue and carry with you to smell throughout the day or add several drops of pure essential oil to a pocket diffuser and use 2-3 times daily.

TOPICALLY

Topical application allows fat-soluble essential oils to be rapidly absorbed and penetrate the membranes of the cells as an effective delivery method to the rest of the body. Through the skin, the essential oils get into the bloodstream where they travel to the target location. Massaging the skin can increase absorption of the oils. Some studies have suggested that areas of skin with a higher concentration of sweat glands and hair follicles have a increased rate of absorption including the soles of the feet, arms, and armpits. Caution should be exercised when using any topical aromatherapy preparations around drug injection sites or areas of the body where transdermal medications are in use (i.e., estrogen or nicotine patches, etc.).

The absorption of certain essential oil chemical compounds has been confirmed through analysis of blood concentrations with maximum levels attained in as little as 10 minutes.

HOW INHALATION WORKS

Inhaled substances pass down the trachea into the bronchi, and from there into finer and finer bronchioles, ending at the microscopic, sac-like alveoli of the lungs, where gaseous exchange with the blood mainly takes place. The alveoli are extremely efficient at transporting small molecules, such as essential oil constituents, into the blood. This efficiency increases with the rate of blood flow through the lungs, the rate and depth of breathing, and with the fat-solubility of the molecules. Essential oil constituents absorbed via inhalation may enter the bloodstream and reach the central nervous system with relative ease.

– Robert Tisserand, Essential Oil Safety 2nd Edition

- **Roll-On** – Place essential oil on heart points on left arm, wrists, feet, and over the heart.
- **Rub On** – Rub 1-2 drops of essential oil on the temples and back of neck several times daily. Or, rub essential oil or essential oil blend on the bottom of feet each evening before bed.
- **Massage** – Massage an essential oil blend (with a carrier oil) for several minutes over the heart and carotid arteries along the neck. Be sure to monitor your blood pressure to see if it drops after massaging oils in. Reapply as desired.

INGESTION

If you are considering ingesting essential oils, you will want to treat your essential oils like powerful medicines, because that is what they are. Taking an oil orally is nearly ten times stronger than when applied topically, so its smart to start with a very small amount and increase gradually. While many essential oils are safe when used internally, some are not. Be sure to read about the oil and do your research to know of any warnings or contradictions. Also, you will want to be aware of proper dosage protocols. The necessary internal dose and frequency is dependent on several factors such as age, size, and health condition which will vary from person to person. One essential oil company states on their website, "The recommended internal dose of essential oils is 1–5 drops, depending on the oil or blend." Taking more than that is not advantageous; in fact, it can be harmful. It is better to take a smaller dose, which can be repeated every 4–6 hours as needed. A low daily dose is recommended for extended internal use.

Only therapeutic quality essential oils should be used when taken internally. Please be sure to check and determine that it is safe for consumption and is GRAS (generally regarded as safe by the FDA). Maximum dosage and the threshold of safe use, whether internal, topical or through inhalation varies based on each individual oil (depending on the chemical structure and metabolism of a substance).

When using essential oils internally doses in the range of one to three drops, one to two times a day (for adults) and are following a protocol appropriate for their health. Caution should be used as all essential oils are not recommended for ingestion. It is recommended that you receive guidance from a qualified health professional before ingesting essential oils. Please store your oils in a safe place away from children.

Using the appropriate amount of essential oil in a vegetable capsule that has been properly diluted can be can be maximally absorbed by the gut for the whole body effect. But like medicines,

GRAS is the Food and Drug Administration's acronym for food additives "Generally Recognized as Safe." FA is the abbreviation for ingredients approved as food additives. Essential oils are included on this list (EO), as many are used for food flavorings and preservatives. The FDA GRAS Inventory list does not include suggested safe dosages, only that items listed are safe in commonly used amounts in order to achieve the necessary effect as a food additive.

essential oil ingestion carries with it the potential for side-effects, mild to severe, including seizures and poisoning.

- **Capsules** – Add one or two drops of essential oil to a "00" gelatin capsule filled with a carrier oil such as olive or coconut oil to buffer the essential oil. Take orally as you would with traditional supplements. A single oil or essential oil blend may be used in this way. For example, a capsule is filled with 20% essential oil diluted with 80% vegetable oil (one ml=20 drops approximately). Each "00" capsule holds approximately 0.7-.91mL or 14 drops, and "0" capsules hold 10 drops of oil. Enteric-Coated Gelatin Capsules could be used as well since they do not release the essential oil until they are in the small intestine.

- **Juice or Water** – Add one or two drops of essential oil to a small glass of juice. Stir to blend well as oil will tend to float on the surface. A solubol can be added as a dispersant to distribute the oils.

- **Tea** – Add one or two drops of essential oil to a ¼ teaspoon of honey and stir into a cup of tea or warm water. Be sure to not overheat the water, as oils will evaporate. Sip slowly.

- **Swishing** – Add several drops of essential oil to a ½ cup of water and swish around the mouth before swallowing.

- **Sugar Cube** – Use a dropper to add one or two drops of essential oil to a cube of sugar. It can be taken directly or added to a drink.

- **Honey** – Essential oils can be blended with honey water. Mix 1-2 drops essential oil into 1 Tsp. honey, add warm water and drink. Or add 1-2 drops of essential oil or essential oil blend to a tablespoon of honey, stir with a toothpick, and take orally.

For adults, the recommended oral dosage with essential oils is 1-3 drops, two to three times a day. Maximum daily dose is 12 drops. *Some essential oil websites recommend up to 20 drops a day, which is quite high and is therefore not recommended.

Some professionals recommend using essential oils two weeks out of the month or taking 1 drop, three times a day for an extended period of time. Others suggest using 1-2 drops, two to three times a day for five days and take two days rest. Either way, it is advisable to take breaks in your essential oil usage.

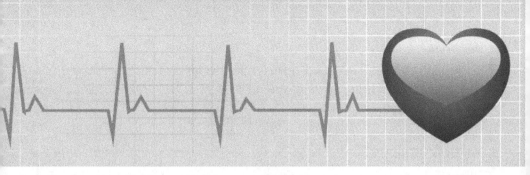

OTHER
METHODS OF USE

GARGLE/MOUTHWASH

Add 2-3 drops of essential oil to 1 teaspoon of water to use as a mouthwash.

BATH

For a full bath, mix 8-10 drops of essential oil into two ounces of sea salts or a cup of milk then pour into a running bath. Agitate water in a figure-eight motion to make sure the oil is mixed well, preventing irritation to mucous membranes.

Another method is to add essential oils after the bath has been drawn. Mix essential oils into a palm full of liquid soap, shampoo or a tablespoon of Jojoba oil and swish around to dissolve in the tub. Soak for 15-20 minutes.

SHOWER

While showering, add a drop or two of essential oil to a washcloth and rub on the body.

MASSAGE

A variety of techniques used in massage therapy can incorporate the use of essential oils. Add 6-9 drops of essential oil to 1 Tablespoon of your favorite carrier oil to massage into body.

LOTIONS/CREAMS

Blending essential oils in an unscented, natural lotion/cream base allow you to benefit from the therapeutic qualities of the essential oil, giving you a non-oily way to apply essential oils. This is especially useful for someone with a skin condition that does not do well with oils. The dilution rate for using essential oils in a lotion base is no more than 2%. For adults, use 20 drops of essential oil to four ounces of lotion. For children and elderly, use 10 drops of essential oil to four ounces of lotion.

SPRAYS/SPRITZERS

Creating your own body sprays and facial mists is one of the easiest ways to use essential oils. For a facial mist, use 8-10 drops of essential oil in a four-ounce spray bottle filled with distilled water. For body sprays, add 20-30 drops of essential oil per four-ounce spray bottle filled with distilled water. For room sprays, use 40-60 drops of essential oil per four-ounce spray bottle with the remainder filled with distilled water.

BODY OILS

Mix 30 drops of essential oil per one ounce of cold-pressed carrier oil such as coconut oil. Choose an all-purpose oil that relieves stress and/or tension, headaches, and smells terrific.

INHALATION

Inhalation can be enhanced with the use of a nebulizer or a cool-mist diffuser in which essential oils are dispersed into the air. Other devices such as a light ring, vaporizer, or electric burner may be used instead, though heating oils may alter their molecular structure and can lose some of their effectiveness.

Inhalation is one of the easiest methods of use and is considered the most direct pathway for an aromatic blend or essence. When inhaled, fragrant vapors enter the lungs and are instantly released into the bloodstream for delivery to every cell in the body. Scientific research shows that essential oils can remain in a person's bloodstream for up to 4-6 hours, depending on the essential oil.

Essential oils that are properly diffused are known to kill bacteria and viruses, improve mental clarity, enhance or calm emotions, and increase feelings of well-being. Over time, oils diffused can strengthen the immune system, reduce mold, and eliminate unpleasant odors. If a diffuser is not available, making a room spray, personal inhaler, or placing a few drops on a tissue to inhale will suffice. All are very effective ways to benefit from the healing properties of essential oils in the treatment of high cholesterol. For inhalation, use intermittent exposure (not more than 15 minutes in an hour).

DIRECT INHALATION

Apply 2-3 drops of essential oils into your hand and rub palms together. Cup hands over the nose and mouth. Inhale vapors deeply several times.

HUMIDIFIER/VAPORIZER

For a humidifier or vaporizer, place 10 drops of essential oil undiluted into the unit.

LINENS/BLANKETS

Add your favorite essential oil to a spray bottle with water and spray to freshen bed sheets and blankets at bedtime and enhance deep sleep.

POTTERY/ELECTRIC BURNERS

A wide range of burners is available to use—some electric, some using tea light candles. Generally, tea light candles are not too hot for diffusing essential oils, but you may want to drop oils over glass stones or add water to the top part to help diffuse fragrance. Use caution around an open fire, as essential oils are flammable. Six drops of oil are recommended for everyday use; however, you may want to reduce the amount of oil used for rooms of the elderly or children.

NEBULIZER/DIFFUSER

Place 25 drops of essential oil undiluted inside the diffuser and use as needed. Limit diffusion of new oils to 10 minutes each day increasing the time until desired effects are reached. Adjust times for different-sized rooms and the strength of each fragrance. Unlike cheap fragrant oils purchased at department stores to mask odors, diffusing pure essential oils actually alters the structure of the molecules that create odors – rendering them harmless. Essential oils increase the available oxygen in the room and produce negative ions, which kill microbes.

QUICK REFERENCE BLENDING CHART

Here's a quick guide to use in determining how much essential oil to use for each application. For recipes and formulas, be sure to follow amounts listed in the directions. For children, elderly and pregnant women, please divide the essential oil amount in half for body applications.

Method	Carrier/Amount	Essential Oils Drops
Vaporizer	Full	5-10
Humidifier	Full	5-10
Steam Inhalation	Full Bowl	2-3
Diffuser/Nebulizer	-	10-25
Tea Lights/Burner	-	4-6
Room Spray	4 ounces	80-100
Body Lotion	4 ounces	25
Body Oil	4 ounces	50
Massage Oil	1 tablespoon	7-10
Shampoo	1 ounce	10
Conditioner	1 ounce	10
Chest Rub	1 ounce	15-25
Tissue	-	1-2
Mouthwash	1 teaspoon	2-3
Foot Bath/Spa	Small Tub	5
Bath	Full Tub	8-10
Shower	Washcloth	1-2

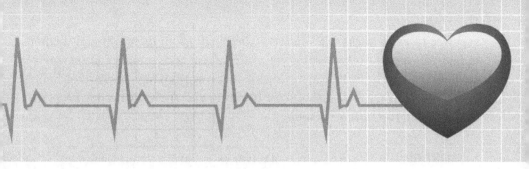

ESSENTIAL OIL RECIPES FOR LOWERING CHOLESTEROL

The following recipes are easy to make and simple to use. Keep in mind, because the root cause of high cholesterol may vary, results may differ from person to person. You will want to experiment and try different essential oils to see which blend is right for you, as no one protocol addresses every situation. You may choose to use one blend in the morning, and another at night. That's fine. Just remember to apply topical blends at least three-four times a day. The key points for application include the wrists, the feet, over the heart, on the carotidal arteries, and along the back of the neck.

The use of certain essential oils such as Lemongrass, Dill, or Bergamot for lowering high cholesterol can be very effective and but may depend on its delivery method.

Feel free to experiment with different combinations of these oils and methods to find which one works best for you. Each oil contains unique and therapeutic qualities that can be beneficial for anyone suffering from high cholesterol. Simply ingest, inhale or massage one of these blends in and allow the healing properties to soothe and revitalize your soul.

SMART TIP: Add a drop or two of Cassia essential oil to your drinking water (on a sugar cube) to help regulate cholesterol.

Some websites suggest taking a daily capsule with 5-6 drops Lemongrass, or Lemongrass with Cypress and Lavender, or Lemongrass with Cassia. For beginners, start with one drop of Clove Bud and 2 drops of Lemongrass twice daily for thirty days. Later, you can add two drops of Grapefruit essential oil to the blend if you choose.

SMART TIP: Add a couple of drops of Cinnamon essential oil with honey and stir into your oatmeal in the morning.

POSSIBLE CAPSULE COMBINATIONS:

British doctors recommend Rosemary oil to their patients with high cholesterol levels. Two to three drops of Rosemary can be taken in a capsule filled with olive oil daily.

Myrrh can be taken by capsule, adding 1-2 drops of essential oil filled with olive oil, twice daily.

One drop of Oregano can be taken by capsule filled with a carrier oil such as olive, twice a day. Basil is another oil used.

Lemongrass, clinically proven to lower cholesterol can be taken internally. Add a drop in a gelatin capsule with olive oil, or place one drop in a teaspoon of honey or a drop in 4 oz. of soy or almond milk. When you're just starting, either take the Lemongrass oil 3 times a day in a capsule or apply it 3 times a day. You may want to cut back to two times a day after checking your cholesterol for results.

Dill can be taken in a vegetable capsule with olive oil.

SMART TIP: Add one or two drops of Grapefruit essential oil to a juice to help flush out toxins from the body.

CHOLESTEROL WELLNESS BLEND

4 drops Clary Sage essential oil

2 drops Cinnamon Bark essential oil

1 drop Helichrysum essential oil

10ml (2 tsp.) Jojoba oil (or another carrier oil such as Apricot)

What to Do:

1. In a small glass bottle or container, add the essential oils.
2. Add the Jojoba carrier oil and shake to blend.
3. Gently rub several drops of the blend into the wrists, the feet, over the heart, along with the carotidal arteries and along the back of the neck after showering in the morning.
4. Apply three times a day (if using this blend throughout the day). Use consistently for at least 30 days. For external use only.

PEACEFUL SLEEP TOPICAL BLEND

3 drops Bergamot essential oil

2 drops Frankincense essential oil

1 drop Ylang Ylang essential oil

15ml (1 tbsp.) Apricot oil (or another carrier oil such as Almond)

What to Do:

1. In a small glass bottle or container, add the essential oils.
2. Add the Apricot carrier oil, replace the cap and shake to blend.
3. Gently rub several drops of the blend into the wrists, the feet, over the heart, along with the carotidal arteries and along the back of the neck after bathing in the evening before bed.
4. Apply three times a day (if using this blend throughout the day).

EVENING STEAM INHALATION BLEND

3 drops Bergamot essential oil

2 drops Lavender essential oil

1 drop Ylang Ylang essential oil

What to Do:
1. In a small bowl add steaming hot water.
2. Place 2-3 drops of essential oil blend into the water and stir to mix.
3. Place a towel over your head and inhale for three to five minutes.

LOVE MY HEART ROLL-ON BLEND

10 drops Lavender essential oil

10 drops Cypress essential oil

10 drops Lemongrass essential oil

10 ml (2 tsp.) Fractionated Coconut oil (or another carrier oil)

What to Do:
1. In a 10ml glass roll-on bottle, add the essential oils.
2. Fill the remaining space with the fractionated coconut oil. Shake to blend.
3. To use, roll the oil blend on the wrists, on the bottoms of the feet, along the neck and over the chest, three times a day.

CHOLESTEROL ROLL-ON BLEND

5 drops Lemongrass essential oil

5 drops Cypress essential oil

5 drops Bergamot essential oil

5 drops Rosemary essential oil

10 ml (2 tsp.) Fractionated Coconut oil (or another carrier oil)

What to Do:

1. In a 10ml glass roll-on bottle, add the essential oils.
2. Fill the remaining space with the fractionated coconut oil. Shake to blend.
3. To use, roll the oil blend on the wrists, on the bottoms of the feet, along the neck and over the chest, two to three times a day.

HOW LOW CAN YOU GO BLEND

2 drops Basil essential oil

2 drops Lemongrass essential oil

2 drops Ginger essential oil

10 drops Coconut carrier oil

What To Do:

1. In a small bottle or container, add all essential oils.
2. Fill the remaining space in the bottle with your favorite carrier oil. Shake to blend.
3. Apply several drops to the bottoms of the feet and massage in. Rub several drops into the wrists, along the breastbone, along the carotidal arteries, and along the back of the neck.

HEATHLY BALANCE ESSENTIAL BLEND

1 drop Lemon essential oil

1 drop Peppermint essential oil

1 drop Black Pepper essential oil

10 drops Favorite carrier oil

What To Do:

1. In the palm of your hand, mix essential oils and carrier oil with your finger.
2. Rub blend into the chest and along the arms. Breathe in deeply.

ANGINA RELIEF BLEND

3 drops Lavender essential oil

3 drops Sweet Marjoram essential oil

3 drops Ylang Ylang essential oil

10 drops Favorite carrier oil

What To Do:

1. In the palm of your hand, mix essential oils and carrier oil with your finger.
2. Rub blend on the soles of your feet and along the carotidal arteries.

CHOLESTEROL BATH BLEND

This meditative blend soothes the mind and quiets the soul.

2 drops Lavender essential oil

2 drops Ylang Ylang essential oil

1 drop Basil essential oil

½ cup Bath Salts (optional)

What To Do:

1. In a small bottle or container add essential oils. Stir to blend.
2. Add several drops of this blend to a running bath and swish to mix thoroughly in water. Or, mix with bath salts first and then add to a hot bath.
3. Relax and inhale the aromas, allowing the oils to penetrate the whole body.

ESSENTIAL SIX BLEND

This blend offers a powerful punch to the cardiovascular system and boosts circulation.

6 drops Peppermint essential oil

4 drops Myrrh essential oil

4 drops Rosemary essential oil

4 drops Cassia essential oil

3 drops Basil essential oil

3 drops Bergamot essential oil

25 drops Coconut oil (or choose your favorite carrier oil from the directory)

What To Do:

1. In a small bottle or container, add all essential oils.
2. Fill the remaining space in the bottle with Coconut oil or another carrier oil. Shake to blend.
3. Apply several drops to the bottoms of the feet and massage in. Rub several drops into the wrists, along the breastbone, along the carotidal arteries, and along the back of the neck.
4. This blend may be added to bath salts and used in a bath, too.

LOVE MY BODY MASSAGE BLEND

Your body works hard for you. Take time to reciprocate your appreciation by offering support and nourishment with a massage using this blend.

4 drops Petitgrain essential oil
4 drops Ylang Ylang essential oil
1 drop Lemongrass essential oil
1 drop Neroli essential oil
1 ounce Favorite carrier oil

What To Do:
1. In a bottle or small container, add essential oils.
2. Fill the remaining space with a carrier oil. Replace cap and shake to blend.
3. Massage into the body or have a massage therapist apply the blend for you.
4. Use daily or as needed.

HEARTWARMING BATH SOAK

Slink down into a warm, relaxing bath and allow your body to absorb these essences of life.

3 drops Coriander essential oil
2 drops Clary Sage essential oil
1 drop Grapefruit essential oil
½ cup Bath Salts (optional)

What To Do:
Stir essential oils into a running bath, or add to bath salts first. Soak in the tub for 15-20 minutes. Repeat daily or as needed.

CHOLESTEROL DIFFUSER BLEND

Make this essential oil blend ahead of time and have ready to use when life gets hectic. Add several drops to a cool-mist diffuser and run for 10-15 minutes twice daily.

2 drops Neroli essential oil
3 drops Lavender essential oil
2 drops Ylang Ylang essential oil
4 drops Bergamot essential oil
Airtight container

What To Do:
1. In a glass bottle, add all of the essential oils. Shake to blend.
2. Add several drops of the essential oil blend into a diffuser at work or in your home and run for 15 minutes in the morning and evening before bedtime. You can also inhale from the bottle to help induce calm.

TAKE IT EASY BLEND

Use this blend to stop heart racing, smooth out muscle tissue, ease spasms and improve circulation.

2 drops Lemongrass essential oil
2 drops Marjoram essential oil
2 drops Cypress essential oil
2 drops Clove Bud essential oil

What To Do:
1. In a glass bottle, add all of the essential oils. Shake to blend.
2. Apply to the chest area around the heart and to the bottoms of the feet in the morning and in the evening.

BALANCE CAPSULE BLEND

This blend can be taken by capsule for lowering cholesterol levels and bringing balance and harmony to your circulation.

1 drops Rosemary essential oil
1 drop Lemon essential oil
1 drop Ginger essential oil
Olive Oil
"00" Empty Capsule

What To Do:

1. Separate the two parts of the capsule. Remove the top half (wider cap). You will only be filling the bottom half.
2. Using a glass dropper, add essential oil one drop at a time directly into the capsule. This needs to be done carefully to not add too many drops or drip oil on the side of the capsule which will make it sticky.
3. Fill the remaining space with olive oil.
4. Take the capsule immediately after filling it. These capsules will begin to dissolve right after filling it.
5. Take one capsule once in the morning and once in the evening.

Tip:
This recipe can be made ahead and stored in a glass bottle with a dropper cap to easily fill capsules as needed.

LOWLEST CAPSULE BLEND #2

Here is a variation of the capsule blend. Naturally, you can substitute essential oils using 1-3 drops of essential oil per capsule.

1 drops Lemongrass essential oil
1 drop Clove Bud essential oil
Olive Oil
"00" Empty Capsule

What To Do:
1. Separate the two parts of the capsule. Remove the top half (wider cap). You will only be filling the bottom half.
2. Using a glass dropper, add essential oil one drop at a time directly into the capsule. This needs to be done carefully to not add too many drops or drip oil on the side of the capsule which will make it sticky.
3. Fill the remaining space with olive oil.
4. Take the capsule immediately after filling it. These capsules will begin to dissolve right after filling it.
5. Take one capsule once in the morning and once in the evening.

Tip:
You can substitute any other the food grade essential oils in this recipe, such as Rosemary for Clove Bud, or Grapefruit essential oil for Lemongrass. There are numerous combinations.

CREATING YOUR OWN BLENDS FOR LOWERING CHOLESTEROL

Coming up with your own essential oil blend for reducing cholesterol levels is easy to do when you follow the blend by note technique. Your essential oil blend will contain one or more oils from each of the above categories: Base note, Middle note, and a Top note (see chart on next page). Some apothecaries recommend using a fourth note, a fixative or bridge notes such as Lavender, Chamomile, Marjoram or Myrrh. The bridge is what helps the other three oils blend together. Oftentimes Vitamin E oil is used for topical blends.

The following chart contains essential oils that are known to be beneficial for high cholesterol. Each essential oil is listed by its common name and note classification: Top, Middle, and Base.

OILS FOR CHOLESTEROL

TOP	MIDDLE	BASE
Bay Laurel	Cassia	Cypress
Basil	Cinnamon	Frankincense
Bergamot	Clove Bud	Ginger
Clary Sage (m)	Coriander	Helichrysum
Grapefruit	Chamomile	Myrrh
Garlic	Dill	Turmeric
Lemon	Goldenrod	Ylang Ylang
Lemongrass	Lavender	
Lime	Marjoram	
Orange	Melissa	
Oregano	Peppermint	
Neroli (m)	Rosemary	
Petitgrain	Sage	
Tangerine		

Some oils made fall into more than one category. This is possible because of the many components essential oils possess and the synergy effect a blend might draw out of that oil. For this reason, you may find aromatherapists disagree to which group they fall in. However, don't let this trouble you. Instead, let this work to your advantage when creating your therapeutic blends. For instance, there may come a time when you have several middle note essential oils on hand to choose from, but no top notes for your particular condition. In this case, you could use an essential oil that may be a top note and middle note as your top note, and choose a different oil as your middle note.

Follow this simply as a guide when orchestrating your blends and let your nose have the final say.

Top Notes are oils that have a light, fresh aroma. It is the first scent you smell after applying a blend to the skin. Although they quickly evaporate, the top note is what gives us our first impression of a blend. Common top notes include Lemon, Bergamot, Orange, Lime and other citrus oils. In fact, Bergamot oil is one of the most widely essential oils used in the perfumery and toiletry industry, together with Neroli and Lavender, as the main ingredients for the classic Eau-de-cologne fragrance.

Most top notes are made up chemically of aldehydes and esters, which are generally found in oils from fruits, flowers, and leaves.

For Therapeutic Blending: Use 3 to 15 drops of a top note per 30 ml (or one ounce) carrier.

Middle Notes, also referred to as heart notes, are usually the inspiration for an aromatic blend and includes floral scents such as Roman Chamomile, Lavender, or Neroli. It is generally considered the heart of the blend as it often serves to cover up any unpleasant scents that may come from the base notes. Essential oils classified as middle notes are sometimes referred to as enhancers, equalizers, or balancers. Chemically, these are monoterpene alcohols found mostly in herbs and leaves. Examples of essential oil middle notes include Lavender, Roman Chamomile, Cypress, Geranium, Juniper Berry, Rosemary, and Peppermint. Middle notes are what we smell when the scent from the top notes fades. This scent often evaporates after 15 seconds. The middle note can last 2-4 hours in the body and as the "heart" of the blend can play on the emotions. Middle notes are often found in flowers, leaves, and needles. They also act to bring together the top and base note as a "synergy" in a blend.

For Therapeutic Blending: Use 2 to 10 drops of a middle note per 30 ml (or one ounce) carrier.

Base Notes, usually the backbone and foundation of the blend, is what the users will remember most about a particular fragrance. The scent of base notes will last the longest in the air and are what you smell after about 30 seconds of applying it to your skin. The base note is added to the mixture first. Examples of essential oil base notes include Vanilla, Sandalwood, Patchouli, Frankincense, Cinnamon, or other earthy and woodsy scents. Typically, a therapeutic blend has only one base note oil in it as it will stay the longest on the skin and can last up to 72 hours in the body. Aromatic blends can have one or more base oils to add character.

Chemically speaking, base notes are made up of sesquiterpenes or diterpenes and are mainly found in roots, gums, and resins. Though therapeutic blends will typically contain one base note while aromatic blends may contain more than one, for any blend to be successful, they must have a combination of all three notes.

For Therapeutic Blending: Use 1 to 5 drops of a base note per 30 ml (or one ounce) carrier.

It is important when making an essential oil blend for your cholesterol to mix the extracts in order starting with the base note, followed by the middle note and finally the top note. This ensures your blend will create an aroma known as a "bouquet" by staying in tune with odor intensity as well as finding notes that strike a chord and harmonize well together in therapeutic properties.

Just remember, for every drop of the base note, you add 2 drops of middle note and 3 drops of the top note. This will ensure that your blend is well-rounded having all three notes, and is chemically balanced between monoterpenes, sesquiterpenes, and phenols.

> **SMART TIP:** Determining which essential oils are best for you to use for your medical issues means looking at all your conditions as a whole and finding the oils that will address as many as possible. Treating your high cholesterol is a good place to start with a therapeutic grade essential oils treatment regimen.

MAKING YOUR FIRST CHOLESTEROL BLEND

Now that you have learned about how many drops of each note to use in your essential oil blend and have checked the precautions, it's time to start blending.

1. Before you begin, gather all of the necessary equipment: bottles, pipettes, essential oils, paper towels, labels, vials, and/or containers.
2. Make sure the counter space is clean, and the area you are working in is well ventilated. You may want to put down wax paper (or a paper towel) to prevent any damage to the countertop from accidental spills. This will also make clean up much easier.
3. If you are using essential oils that are new to you, place one drop of the oil on a test strip (or small piece of paper) and wave it under your nose. Inhale the fragrance. If this fragrance is not what you had in mind, choose another oil and test again. You will want to do this with each oil until you have settled on the ones you want to use for your blend. It is a good idea to have a can of coffee grounds to smell after each fragrance to clear your palette.

4. Once, you have chosen the three oils for your blend, wave all three test strips fanned out beneath your nose and see if you like it. You may not care too much, as long as it helps lower your cholesterol, but keep in mind, if you despise the scent, you may be hesitant about using it regularly.

5. Check the safety precautions for the essential oils you have chosen to make sure there aren't any contradictions. Always take into consideration any other health conditions such as epilepsy, or any medications that may cause an adverse effect. The safety precautions must always be taken into consideration for the method you choose in their usage and for the person you are formulating the blend for.

6. Choose a new, clean bottle to use. Using a pipette, extract each essential oil into the bulb to place in your bottle. You may need to squeeze more than once to get the amount you want. Remember to use a separate pipette or glass eye dropper for each of the oils used.

   Add your base note essential oil first, one drop at a time. This is typically the most vicious or thickest oil. Next, add the middle note essential oil, followed by the top note essential oil. Be careful to use only the exact number of drops your recipe calls for. One drop too many can alter the results. Replace the cap on the bottle and shake to mix oils together.

7. Add your essential oil blend to a carrier oil (or lotion, gel, sea salts, etc.) and blend well to distribute the oils. What you use as your carrier and how much to add will depend on which method of application (Massage Blend, Bath Blend, Room Spray, etc.) you choose.

TIP: Always leave ½ inch of head space at the top of your bottle allowing your pure essential oil blend to breathe and expand.

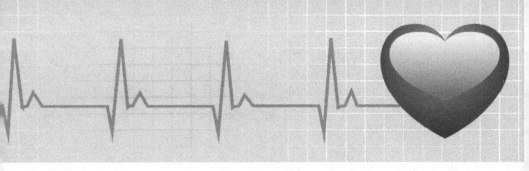

BASIC RECIPES FOR YOUR CHOLESTEROL BLENDS

Now that you have a basic understanding of how to blend essential oils together for high cholesterol levels follow these simple recipes as a guideline for preparing your own products. You can formulate your own blend that will deliver the healing benefits you are seeking using three of the essential oils on the recommended list.

The recipes below are based on blending by notes. Of course, there is plenty of room for creativity as there are no hard and fast rules when it comes to creating your individual blend. You can add more or less. Feel free to change these to suit your own personal taste!

BASIC MASSAGE OIL BLEND RECIPE

Here is an easy-to-follow basic recipe for making a massage blend! You get to decide which essential oils to use depending on the type of massage and affect you looking to achieve.

What You Will Need:

1 ounce (30 ml) Carrier Oil, Lotion, or Gel
9-15 drops Top Note Essential Oil
6-10 drops Middle Note Essential Oil
3-5 drops Base Note Essential Oil
Plastic Bottle

What To Do:

1. Pour your carrier oil, lotion or gel into a clean bottle.

2. Add your essential oils one drop at a time, starting with your base note, followed by the middle note, and then the top note.

3. Shake well to mix oils and carrier together.

4. Add a label with name, ingredients, and date created.

5. Use two to three times a day.

BASIC BATH GEL BLEND RECIPE

Bath blends are easy to create using this basic recipe with a few essential oils!

What You Will Need:
1 teaspoon Glycerin, Gel, or Aloe Vera
3-12 drops Top Note Essential Oil
2-8 drops Middle Note Essential Oil
1-4 drops Base Note Essential Oil
Small Dish or Bowl

What To Do:
1. In a small dish or bowl, add the glycerin or gel as your fixative.
2. Add your essential oils one drop at a time to the fixative and stir well.
3. Pour your bath blend into a stream of warm running bath water. Enjoy!

Tip:
Always check precautions – especially for essential oils that may cause sensitivity to the skin. Be sure to use a 1% dilution or less with children.

BASIC BODY LOTION BLEND RECIPE

Do you want to try a good body lotion recipe? Why not make your own by following these simple instructions?

What You Will Need:

4 ounces Unscented Lotion, Hydrosol and/or carrier oil
18 drops Top Note Essential Oil
12 drops Middle Note Essential Oil
6 drops Base Note Essential Oil
Plastic Bottle or container

What To Do:

1. Place your carrier oil and/or lotion in your bottle.
2. Add essential oils starting with your base note essential oil first, followed by the middle note, and then the top note essential oil.
3. Recap and shake well to mix.
4. Use two to three times a day.

BASIC LINEN SPRAY BLEND RECIPE

Use this special blend to ease insomnia and ensure better sleep at night. Don't forget when using essential oils for your spray to make sure the ones you choose are relaxing!

What You Will Need:

8 ounces Hydrosol, Floral Water, or Distilled Water

1 Tablespoon Glycerin

60 drops Top Note Essential Oil

40 drops Middle Note Essential Oil

20 drops Base Note Essential Oil

Glass or Plastic Spray Bottle

What To Do:

1. In a clean spray bottle, add the fixative (Glycerin).
   Add your essential oil to the fixative, starting with the base note, followed by the middle note, and then the top note. Shake well.
   Pour the Hydrosol or floral water into the bottle and shake to mix contents well.

2. Spray on bedspread and linens before making the bed.

BASIC BATH SALTS BLEND RECIPE

For this basic bath salts recipe, you can use Dead Sea, Himalayan, or Epsom salts. Soak in a bath with this great blend to soothe away the stress of the day. Your bath salts can be made in advance and stored in a pretty container for convenience.

What You Will Need:

2 cups Epsom Salts

1 cup Sea Salts

1 cup Baking Soda

30 drops Top Note Essential Oil

20 drops Middle Note Essential Oil

10 drops Base Note Essential Oil

Wide Mouth Jar or container

What To Do:

1. In a container, add your essential oils starting with the base note, followed by the middle note, and then the top note. Stir to mix well.

2. Add sea salts and mix well to saturate the salts with the oils thoroughly.

3. In a running bath, add bath salts and swish around in the tub to mix thoroughly.

Tip:

Be sure to check precautions for oils that may cause sensitivity to skin. Not recommended for children.

BASIC SALT SCRUB BLEND RECIPE

Salt scrubs are great for increasing circulation. For this basic salt scrub recipe, you can choose which salt you prefer such as Dead Sea, Himalayan, or Epsom salts. Try it for painful joints and achy muscles, too. Your salt scrub can be made fresh each time, or you may want to make some up and store in a cute container for when the time is right.

What You Will Need:

½ cup Sea Salts

2-4 ounces Carrier Oil (your choice)

9-12 drops Top Note Essential Oil

6-8 drops Middle Note Essential Oil

3-4 drops Base Note Essential Oil

Wide Mouth Jar or container

What To Do:

1. In a container, add your carrier oil, such as Almond or Coconut oil. Add your essential oils starting with the base note, followed by the middle note, and then the top note. Stir to mix well.

2. Add sea salts and mix well to saturate the salts with the oils thoroughly.

3. In the shower or bath, scrub the salt solution into the skin in upward motions toward the heart and in the direction of the lymph flow.

Tip:

Be sure to check precautions for oils that may cause sensitivity to skin. Not recommended for children.

BASIC SALVE BLEND RECIPE

Carrying a small tin in your pocket is not only convenient but is easy to use.

What You Will Need:
½ – 1 cup Olive Oil or another Carrier Oil
2 teaspoons Beeswax
9 drops Top Note Essential Oil
6 drops Middle Note Essential Oil
3 drops Base Note Essential Oil
Small Jar or Tin

What To Do:
1. Using a double glass boiler, heat the oil over hot water. If you prefer, you can heat oil in a pan directly over the burner on low heat or in a microwave until warm.
2. Add the beeswax and stir until melted.
3. Let oil cool slightly (not too long or it will set up).
4. Add the essential oils, starting with the base note, followed by the middle note, then the top note. Stir to blend.
5. Pour mixture into jars or tins immediately. If mixture begins to set, just reheat slightly.

Tip:
For variation, you can use solid Coconut oil and omit the beeswax. You may also want to add 6-8 Vitamin E oil capsules as a preservative.

BASIC BATH TEA BLEND RECIPE

For an extraordinary bathing experience, try adding dried herbs and flower petals to your running bath for a relaxing time!

What You Will Need:

2 cups Herbs (Lavender flowers, Mint leaves, etc.)

1 cup Sea Salts (your choice)

6 drops Top Note Essential Oil

4 drops Middle Note Essential Oil

2 drops Base Note Essential Oil

What To Do:

1. In a mixing bowl, add dried herbs and flower petals to sea salts and stir to blend.

2. Add essential oils starting with the base oil, followed by the middle note, then finally the top note. Stir to mix well.

3. Store in an airtight container or jar. Add a scoopful of the mixture into a cotton or linen bag and hang under running bath water. If you do not have a bag, add mixture directly into bath. Enjoy!

BASIC BODY DETOX WRAP BLEND RECIPE

Body wraps are a popular way to lose weight and fight cellulite, which in turn helps lower cholesterol. In addition, you can kick start your body's immune system by ridding yourself of accumulated chemicals and toxins stored in the body's lymphatic system.

What You Will Need:
3 ounces Distilled Water
12 drops Top Note Essential Oil
6 drops Middle Note Essential Oil
3 drops Base Note Essential Oil
Small Glass Spray Bottle
Plastic Wrap

What To Do:
1. In a small spray bottle, add your essential oils starting with the base note, followed by the middle note, then the top note oil. Add the distilled water to the bottle, close and shake to blend.
2. Spray a bath towel thoroughly with the detox blend. Wrap the towel around your body, followed by tightly wrapping plastic wrap around yourself. Relax for 20 minutes before removing plastic wrap and towel.

BASIC ROLL-ON OIL BLEND RECIPE

This basic recipe can be used to create a roll-on bottle applicator for your essential oil blend, depending on the oils you have on hand. Keep track of what you add or change, so you'll know how to make your favorite blends at a later time.

What You Will Need:

½ Ounce Jojoba Oil

9 drops Top Note Essential Oil

6 drops Middle Note Essential Oil

3 drops Base Note Essential Oil

Dark Bottle

What To Do:

1. Add your carrier oil such as Jojoba to a clean, dark glass bottle.

2. When adding essential oils, start with the base note and then add the middle note, followed by the top note. As you add each one, check the scent to make sure it is what you are looking for.

3. Insert the ball insert and apply 2-3 times a day.

BASIC BATH OIL BLEND RECIPE

After a long day, soaking in a warm bath with a relaxing essential oil blend can be a delightful treat. Not only does it help take the edge off tense muscles, but it also ensures a better night's sleep. For early risers, starting your day with an invigorating essential oil blend at bath time may be more your speed, kick-starting your morning! Of course, a bath essential oil blend for achy joints can be helpful any time of day!

What You Will Need:

1 cup Almond Oil or Coconut Oil

30 drops Top Note Essential Oil

20 drops Middle Note Essential Oil

10 drops Base Note Essential Oil

Corked container

Crystal beads, dried flowers, small seashells, etc. (Optional)

What To Do:

1. Pour the carrier oil through a funnel into the corked container, leaving about an inch at the top.

2. When adding essential oils, start with the base note and then add the middle note, followed by the top note. As you add each one, check the scent to make sure it is what you are looking for.

3. Cork the container and agitate the bottle gently.

4. Let it sit for 2-3 days before using. Add decor to your bottle.

5. For use, pour ½ – 1 teaspoon into the palm of your hand and gently massage into the body after a bath.

BASIC NASAL INHALER BLEND RECIPE

Filling a new nasal inhaler with your personal essential oil blend is an effective way to experience the therapeutic power of essential oils when suffering from high cholesterol or emotional issues. Inhalers are also great to use for colds, flu, headaches, allergies, lung and chest congestion. They are small enough to carry in a pocket or purse and have on hand for immediate relief. Add 15-18 drops of your essential oil blend to your inhaler.

What You Will Need:

9 drops Top Note Essential Oil

6 drops Middle Note Essential Oil

3 drops Base Note Essential Oil

Glass or Plastic Disposable Dropper

Small Plastic Inhaler

What To Do:

1. In a small bottle, add essential oils starting with the base oil, followed by the middle note, then finally the top note. Stir to mix well.
2. Use a glass or disposal dropper to fill nasal inhaler.
3. Carry and take a whiff as needed.

BASIC FOOT OIL BLEND RECIPE

A luxurious foot treatment with essential oils can readily deliver healing throughout the body. The sensitive skin and tissues of the feet take a lot of abuse and deserve a special blend that can easily be massaged in.

What You Will Need:

1 ounce (30ml) Almond Oil

3 drops Top Note Essential Oil

2 drops Middle Note Essential Oil

1 drop Base Note Essential Oil

Plastic or Glass Bottle

What To Do:

1. In a glass or plastic bottle, add your essential oils starting with the base note, followed by the middle note and then the top note. Mix well.

2. Add the Almond oil or another carrier oil to the bottle, replace lid and shake to blend.

3. To use, massage oil blend into feet after a bath or shower, or before bed. Wear soft, cotton socks to bed.

BASIC CAPSULE BLEND

Here is a simple recipe for making an essential oil capsule for ingestion. It is one of the best ways to take essential oils internally and bypass any unpleasant tastes. You an use 1-2 drops of essential oil per capsule (depending on size).

1-2 drops GRAS Essential Oil (20%)
Carrier Oil (80%)

What To Do:
1. Separate the two parts of the capsule. Remove the top half (wider cap). You will only be filling the bottom half.
2. Using a glass dropper, add essential oil one drop at a time directly into the capsule. This needs to be done carefully to not add too many drops or drip oil on the side of the capsule which will make it sticky.
3. Fill the remaining space with olive, coconut, pomegranate, etc.
4. Take the capsule immediately after filling it. These capsules will begin to dissolve right after filling it.
5. Take one capsule once in the morning and once in the evening, or as prescribed by your health practionier.

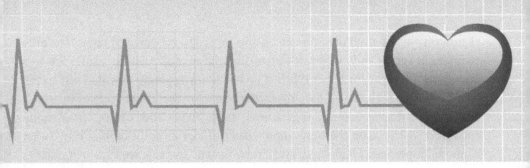

WHICH CARRIER OILS
TO USE

When you use essential oils, in most cases you will want to dilute with a carrier or vegetable oil. Carrier oils come from nuts, seeds or kernels that contain essential fatty acids, fat-soluble vitamins, minerals and other crucial nutrients. You will find a variety of carrier oils to choose from, each possessing different therapeutic properties.

The two primary methods of producing carrier oil are cold-pressed and maceration. These processes ensure they have not been modified by heat, which would destroy the vital nutrients contained in the oil, and are as natural and unadulterated as possible.

Macerated oils, such as calendula and carrot oils, are made from a combination of a base oil such as sunflower and plant material that has been left in an airtight container over a period of time in order to infuse the liquid with the plant's constituents.

Carrier oils and infused oils are used to dilute essential oils and absolutes by offering the necessary lubrication and moisture to the skin for aromatherapy.

Distinct from essential oils, carrier oils do not contain aromatic scents (or only a very faint scent) and evaporate due to their large molecular structure. For this reason, most consider carrier oils just a vehicle for applying essential oils to the skin in massage. However, they do offer their own healing properties in which essential oils do not possess. Your aromatherapy experience can be significantly enhanced by choosing the best combination of carrier and essential oils. Sweet Almond, Sunflower, Hempseed, and Fractionated Coconut are excellent choices to use.

SMART TIP: A massage oil blend with a mixture of 10-15% essential oil and 85-90% carrier oil will ensure a powerful massage oil that is smooth and great-smelling.

SHELF LIFE OF CARRIER OILS

A carrier oil's shelf life, which is the length of time before a particular oil begins to turn rancid, can be greatly influenced by heat and light. You will want to store your oils in a cool, dark place to preserve their freshness, and in some cases refrigerate (e.g. Not Avocado), as heat and sunlight can shorten their shelf life. When refrigerating, oils may appear cloudy but will regain their transparent state upon returning to room temperature. If you have a large amount of carrier oil on hand, you can freeze the unused portion until ready for use.

TIP: Try not to mix too much of your favorite massage blend in advance if you don't plan on using it right away.

Carrier Oil	Shelf Life
Fractionated Coconut	Indefinite
Flaxseed	3-6 months
Grapeseed	3-6 months (up to 9 months, if refrigerated)
Olive	12-18 months
Sweet Almond	12 months
Jojoba	Indefinite
Apricot Kernel	6-12 months
Argan	24 months
Avocado	12 months
Borage	6 months
Carrot Seed	12 months
Cocoa Butter	3-5 years
Coconut (virgin)	2-4 years
Cranberry Seed	2 years
Evening Primrose	6-12 months
Hemp Seed	12 months
Macadamia	12 months
Palm	24 months
Pomegranate Seed	12 months
Rosehip Seed	6 months
Safflower	24 months
Sesame Seed	4-6 months
Shea Butter	Indefinite
Sunflower	12 months
Walnut	12 months
Pumpkin Seed	6-12 months
Meadowfoam Seed	Indefinite
Wheat Germ	1 year

Instead of thinking of carrier oils as merely the method of applying essential oils, explore the unique qualities of carrier oils separately to find the best oil for lowering cholesterol. You can enhance your benefits by using specific essential oils with carriers that actually increase their medicinal qualities. For this reason, consideration will be given to how plant-derived oils deliver health from the outside in. Externally applied oils help the body maintain vital functions in unique ways through both chemical changes and mechanical assistance.

Most carrier oils are unsaturated fats. Saturated fats have carbon bonds that do not bind to other carbon atoms. These oils are solid at room temperature and include animal-derived fats and some plant-derived fats as well. Coconut oil is a saturated fat that is often used as a carrier oil. Fractionated coconut, another common carrier oil, occurs when a coconut molecule has been altered to keep it in a liquid, rather than solid, state. The healing qualities of the oil are not compromised, and the oil can be used the same way a seed or nut oil is used.

When considering vegetable oils for use in capsules, many have the essential fatty acids Omega-6 (linoleic acid) and Omega-3 (linolenic). Essential fatty acids must be acquired through outside sources, primarily through diet, and are critical to maintaining health. According to Aromatherapist Salvatore Battaglia, Omega-6, which is vital for skin, hair, liver function, joints, healing wounds, and circulation, is especially powerful in Evening Primrose oil, a popular and versatile carrier oil. Omega-3 is also in many carrier oils. Taken internally, it helps with vision, muscles, and growth. It is found in fish and some vegetable oils, like linseed and canola. It is known to help circulation, assist in heart health, lower cholesterol and blood pressure, and prevent inflammation. The most important thing to remember about lipid structure in carrier oils is that choosing high-quality, nutritious oils will significantly assist in its vital functions.

Carrier oils are primarily derived from nuts and seeds. They are extracted via cold-pressed technology, meaning high heat is not used. Once oils reach temperatures exceeding 160 degrees Celsius, their structure is altered, making them trans-fats, a kind of mutated fat that the body cannot assimilate properly. Expeller pressing is another common extraction method. By placing seeds or nuts in an expeller, the precious oil is pressed out and then bottled. Superior carrier oils are mechanically pressed oils and have not been subjected to chemical changes.

When carrier oils are used with essential oils topically, they provide a mechanism for the volatile oils to be transported more effectively. Most essential oils when applied externally move through the body system in an hour. A carrier oil, which is thicker than a volatile oil, "holds" the essential oil in place, delivering longer-lasting healing. You want to include the specific healing benefits of carrier oils in your aromatherapy applications as well; it might be useful to look at how carrier oils are sometimes categorized.

Essential oils in aromatherapy are highly concentrated and potent. Although there are only a few exceptions to using essential oils 'neat' or undiluted (such as Lavender and Chamomile), it is ideal always to use a carrier oil with your essential oils to avoid having an adverse effect or skin irritation.

Carrier oils provide the much-needed lubrication, allowing hands to move freely over the skin, helping with the absorption of essential oils into the body. Choose a carrier oil that is light, non-sticky and that can effectively penetrate the skin. Always check the label to make sure it's 100% pure, unrefined and cold-pressed.

CARRIER OILS DIRECTORY

With the vast selection of carrier oils, each with various therapeutic benefits, choosing one will depend on the area it's being applied to, the treatment plan, and any skin sensitivities. When using an oil for massage, the viscosity is an important consideration. Some carrier oils may work better than others in certain applications. For example, Grapeseed oil is generally very thin while Olive oil is much thicker, and others such as Sunflower and Sweet Almond have viscosities halfway between these extremes. You can easily blend carrier oils to combine their properties of viscosity, absorption rate, and benefits. Don't forget to take into consideration the color of your carrier oil when creating a particular recipe where it may affect the outcome of the product; otherwise, for general blending purposes the color of your carrier oil won't matter.

TIP: When shopping for a good quality carrier oil, be sure it's cold-pressed so that all of its natural qualities have been retained.

Almond Oil is one of the most useful, practical and moderately priced carrier oils available. It is ideal for all skin types as it moisturizes and reconditions the skin with its satiny smooth texture. This pale yellow oil quickly absorbs into the skin, leaving your skin feeling soft and non-greasy. Sweet Almond provides relief from itching, soreness, dryness, inflammation, and is especially beneficial for eczema. As a lightly nutty refined oil rich in fatty acids, proteins and Vitamin D, it is everyone's favorite massage base oil for loosening stiff muscles and achy joints.

Dilution: Can be used at 100%.

Apricot Kernel Oil is pale yellow in color and has a light texture, is easily absorbed and moisturizes both the body and face well. Extracted from the kernel of apricot fruit, it contains Vitamin E, which is particularly suitable for mature skin. Vitamins A and B help in healing and rejuvenating skin cells. It is suitable for all skin types, especially for sensitive, inflamed and dry skin. Apricot seeds are well known for the presence of amygdalin, as well as Vitamin B-17 and laetrile, which is a compound considered to have the potential to kill cancer cells without causing any damage to surrounding healthy cells, and lower blood pressure. Studies reveal that the consumption of apricot seeds helped in the lowering of both systolic and diastolic blood pressure in people with high blood pressure.

Dilution: Can be used at 100% or as a blend with other carrier oils such as Sweet Almond oil for a massage at 10% dilution.

Argan Oil comes from Morocco with over 80% unsaturated fatty acids and essential fats. It contains high amounts of Vitamin E and is extremely resistant to oxidation. This cold-pressed oil is considered a treat for mature skin and valued for its nutritive, cosmetic and medicinal properties. Researchers have concluded daily consumption of Argan oil can help prevent various cancers, cardiovascular disease, and obesity. According to the British Journal of Nutrition n (2004), 92, 921–929, "Argan (Argania spinosa) oil lowers blood pressure and improves endothelial dysfunction in spontaneously hypertensive rats." Its medicinal uses also include rheumatism and healing burns. Argan oil is sometimes mixed with Pomegranate Seed oil due to its anti-oxidizing properties.

Dilution: Can be used at 100% or diluted with other carrier oils such as Rosehip Seed, Coconut or Apricot Kernel as a blend.

Avocado Oil is rich in lecithin, Vitamins, A, B1, B2, D, and E. It also contains amino acids, sterols, pantothenic acid, and lecithin. It is known to delay aging as it is rich in essential fatty acids. Avocado quickly penetrates the skin, acts as a sunscreen and helps in cell regeneration. For skin that has been exposed to the sun, mix zinc oxide in half a bottle of Avocado oil and apply. Avocado is greatly praised for those who suffer from skin problems such as eczema, psoriasis, and other skin disorders. The antioxidants and beta-sitosterol found in avocados help to reduce the risk of heart disease and cancer while maintaining eye health in aging adults. Avocados are also rich in monounsaturated fats, which help balance cholesterol levels. An essential nutrient for bone and cardiovascular health, the magnesium found in an avocado is also known to reduce migraines and prevent type II diabetes. The Omega-3 Fatty Acids in avocados may reduce inflammation, high cholesterol, high blood pressure, depression, and arthritis.

Dilution: Can be used at 100%, although in most cases, it is best mixed with another carrier oil such as Sweet Almond or Grapeseed oil to make up 10-30% of the carrier blend.

Borage Seed Oil is naturally one of the greatest sources of GLA or gamma-linolenic acid. It improves the skin texture when used topically. Borage Seed is excellent for use with children with atopic dermatitis. During the Middle Ages, borage was a traditional anti-inflammatory agent used to treat rheumatism and heart disease.

Dilution: Can be utilized at 100% as your carrier oil base, although it is recommended to use with other carrier oils up to 25% for therapeutic applications.

Carrot Seed Oil is rich in beta-carotene, and Vitamins A, B, C, D, and E. This oil is known to heal dry, chapped skin, balance the moisture in the skin and condition the hair, as well. It is suitable for all skin types, especially for dry, mature skin, and is effective for face and neck treatments in reducing wrinkles. Many users find it helpful for burns, wounds, cuts, and scars. Carrot Seed oil contains up to 13 percent alpha-pinene and up to 18 percent carotol. Other contents include daucol, limonene, beta-bisabolene, eugenol, vanillin, various terpenoids, coumarin, and palmitic and butyric acids. The website Drugs.com credits Carrot Seed oil with smooth-muscle relaxant action, as well as the ability to protect the liver, dilate blood vessels and lower blood pressure in animal studies. Carrot Seed absorbs easily into the skin and is excellent for eczema, psoriasis, and itchy scalp.

Dilution: Can be used at 100% or blended with another carrier oil at 10-25%.

Cocoa Butter is a rich and creamy butter (not a carrier oil) that must be warmed to make it liquid. It is an excellent addition to skin care products due to its high level of polyphenols, vitamins, and nutrients. It smoothes, hydrates, and balances skin while providing collagen to support mature skin. Its warm aroma of cocoa is a delightful addition to lotions and creams. Cocoa butter is widely used as a treatment for pregnancy stretch marks. With its A, B1, B2, B3, C, and E vitamins, it is an excellent moisturizer for skin health. Scientists have linked the cocoa (in dark chocolate and cocoa butter) to a reduction of blood pressure and heart disease. According to the American Heart Association, a 2006 study called "Circulation: Heart Failure" reported that middle-aged and elderly women who regularly ate a small amount of chocolate had a 32 percent lower risk of heart failure. Although scientists are not sure why, it may be due to its oleic acid or its cocoa mass polyphenol (CMP), which may protect against heart disease.

Dilution: Its firm texture makes it difficult to work in and needs to be blended with other oils to be workable. Use at a 10% dilution.

Coconut Oil (Fractionated) seems to be quickly becoming the carrier oil of choice because of its broad use in alternative medicine and healing. While it is fractionated, no change has been made chemically. Rather, its molecular structure 'fraction' has been separated, allowing it to remain liquid at room temperature making it much more useful in aromatherapy. Coconut oil is perfect as a moisturizer for the body and conditions brittle, dry or dull hair. Because of its many health benefits, Coconut oil, when used correctly, can prove beneficial in a regimen designed to lower blood pressure. Its light, easily absorbable texture gives skin a smooth satin effect with virtually no scent of its own and an indefinite shelf life. Coconut oil is 92% saturated fat and contains Omega-3 fatty acids, and is believed to be better for lowering blood pressure than other vegetable oils. Omega-3 fatty acids are known to widen your blood vessels and relieve inflammation of the arteries.

Dilution: Can be used at 100%.

Coconut Oil (Virgin) has an incredible balance of natural saturated fatty acids with antibacterial and antiviral properties not found in other oils. Coconut oil is perfect as a skin conditioner for nearly all skin conditions and is believed to stimulate hair growth. It has a light, aromatic coconut scent that becomes solid at room temperature. For this reason, it is recommended to blend with other carrier oils in your body care products. It is fully digestible and is considered a healthy cooking oil. Several virgin coconut oils are high in antioxidants which are positively associated with reducing oxidative stress, and thus lowering blood pressure.

Dilution: Can be used alone directly but is recommended to use 10-25% dilution with other carrier oils.

Cranberry Seed Oil is rich in Vitamin E and A, Omega-3, 6, and 9 fatty acids not available in other carrier oils. This fruity medium texture oil can help reduce signs of aging and heal scars and skin conditions such as eczema and psoriasis. Cranberries are high in antioxidants that help fight free radicals. The oil from the cranberry seed contains high levels of polyunsaturated and monounsaturated fatty acids, phospholipids, phytosterols and huge amounts of antioxidants that offer a variety of health benefits. Cranberries are a good source of phenolic phytochemicals, including phenolic acids. According to an article published in the November 2007 issue of Nutrition Reviews, "Polyphenols found in cranberries may reduce the risk of cardiovascular disease by impeding platelet aggregation, lowering blood pressure and promoting resistance of low-density lipoprotein, or LDL, against oxidation."

Dilution: Can be used at 100%.

Evening Primrose Oil makes a delightful addition to your carrier oil blends. It is the perfect, lightly refined oil that can be used to moisturize, soften and soothe away dry and irritated skin and help with premature aging. Evening primrose contains gamma-linolenic acid, Omega-3 essential fats as well as other fatty acids that help the body produce Prostaglandin E1, which reduces inflammation and improves digestion. Because evening primrose oil contains Omega-6 essential fatty acids that are necessary for good health, it has been known to lower blood pressure. This oil can be taken internally. Please note this oil can go rancid quickly.

Dilution: Due to its cost, it is usually blended with other carrier oils at 10% dilution.

Flaxseed Oil is an emollient, high in essential fatty acids, Vitamin E, B, and minerals. It contains the alpha-linoleic acids (ALAs), which may contribute to lowering blood pressure. Flaxseed is reputed as being an excellent treatment for eczema and psoriasis. It is also known for its anti-inflammatory properties and for preventing scarring and stretch marks. Flaxseed oil contains both Omega-3 and Omega-6 fatty acids, which are needed for health. Flaxseed oil contains the essential fatty acid alpha-linolenic acid (ALA), which the body converts into eicosapentaenoic acid (EPA) and docosahexaenoic acid (DHA), the Omega-3 fatty acids found in fish oil according to the University of Maryland Medical Center's website. ALA may reduce heart disease risks through a variety of ways, including making platelets less "sticky," reducing inflammation, promoting blood vessel health, and lessen the risk of arrhythmia (irregular heart beat). Several human studies also suggest that diets rich in Omega-3 fatty acids (including ALA) may lower blood pressure. This golden oil will leave a greasy feeling on the skin, so it is recommended to add to other carrier oils for use in skincare products.

Dilution: Due to its heavy scent and texture, use at 10% dilution with another carrier oil or carrier oil blend.

Grapeseed Oil is a pleasing, light green and odorless oil, good as a base oil for many creams, lotions and as a carrier oil. Grapeseed oil is pressed from the seeds of a grape and contains OPCs, flavonoids, vitamin E, resveratrol, and fatty acids. It is non-allergenic and has very high levels of linoleic acid, with traces of proanthocyanidins, which are very potent antioxidants. It is reportedly helpful to reduce stretch marks. It is used as an alternative treatment for conditions such as diabetes, hemorrhoids, cancers, high cholesterol, edema, and high blood pressure. A study conducted at the University of California at Davis found that grape seed extract helped control blood pressure. It is especially beneficial for all skin types because of its natural non-allergenic properties. Grapeseed works well, especially when other oils do not absorb well, without leaving a greasy feeling after application. Slightly astringent, it tightens and tones the skin and alleviates acne. Grapeseed makes an ideal carrier oil for body massage bases. Saturation takes longer than some other carrier oils.

Dilution: Can be used at 100%.

Hemp Seed Oil is a hidden treasure of fatty acids, including ALA and GLA, that makes it possibly one of the most nourishing oils available. An analysis shows it contains linoleic acid, Alpha and Gamma Linolenic Acid (omega-6), Palmitic acid, Stearic acid and oleic acid. These essential fatty acids help ward off various age-related diseases and osteoarthritis. Hemp oil has been scientifically proven to improve dermatitis symptoms, reduce blood clots and high blood pressure. Like Evening Primrose, it is supportive of reducing inflammation, which makes it useful for arthritis and autoimmune disorders. It also stimulates hair and nail growth and makes a superb skin moisturizer. Hemp oil contains many healing and regenerative properties and may be applied topically to restore vital organs, as well as skin conditions. Research shows it is beneficial in reducing blood clots and high blood pressure. This rich, slightly green, nutty flavored oil can be taken internally but should be refrigerated.

Dilution: Can be used at 100% or blended with other carrier oils at 20% dilution for massage purposes.

Jojoba Oil is bright and golden in color and is known as one of the best oils (actually a liquid wax) for hair and skin. It penetrates the skin quickly and is excellent for skin nourishment and for healing inflamed skin, psoriasis, eczema, or any sort of dermatitis. Jojoba controls acne and oily skin and makes a terrific scalp cleanser as excess sebum dissolves in Jojoba. It is suitable for all skin types and promotes a healthy, glowing complexion by gently unclogging the pores and lifting embedded impurities. It makes a good base oil for treating rheumatism and arthritis because of its anti-inflammatory actions. Jojoba is suitable for all aromatherapy uses other than a full-body massage. And, because of the oil's antioxidants, it does not become rancid and can even prevent rancidity in other oils.

Dilution: Can be used at 100% but due to its price, many use a 10% dilution with other carrier oils.

Macadamia Oil has a rich golden color with mild nutty undertones. It is made up of 80% monounsaturated fatty acids including oleic acid, Palmitoleic acid, linoleic acid and linolenic acid. This oil's fatty acid closely resembles human sebum, and a recent study shows that the presence of palmitoleic acid plays an active role in the slowing down of lipid peroxidation, thus offering cell protection function. Macadamia provides the skin with a silky feel and is quickly absorbed leaving a smooth, non-greasy feeling. Studies by the Journal of Nutrition revealed that consumption of macadamia nuts lowers plasma total and LDL cholesterol levels in hypercholesterolemic men. It is sensitive to light and will go rancid as a result. Use this oil in small quantities as the scent may overpower the blend.

Dilution: Use at 10-25% dilution with another carrier oil or carrier oil blend.

Meadowfoam Seed Oil with its pale yellow color and medium viscosity makes a nice carrier for many aromatherapy applications. Its rejuvenating properties make it a popular choice for cosmetics and skin care products, especially for its UV protection properties. It is an essential ingredient in many different products such as suntan lotion, massage oils and lotions, hand/facial creams, hair and scalp products, cuticle repair cream, foundations, rouges, face powders, lipsticks, shampoos, and shaving creams. Its rich antioxidant content of Vitamin E, oleic acid (Omega-9 fatty acid), erucic acid, eicosanoic acid, linolenic acid (Omega-6 fatty acid), delta linolenic acid and alpha Omega-3 fatty acids makes it a highly stable oil with an indefinite shelf life. At closer examination, the seed contains useful components such as tocopherol, the primary component of Vitamin E that is known to keep the skin from aging, protects different organs of the body and slows down its degeneration. It also contains docosadienoic acid, which is a polyunsaturated fat known for the benefits that it gives to the heart. Specifically, it can lower cholesterol and triglycerides in the body as well as lower blood pressure.

Dilution: Can be used at 10% dilution with another carrier oil or carrier oil blend.

Olive Oil (Extra Virgin) is light to medium green in color, with a rather dense texture. It is very soothing and carries disinfecting and healing properties. Olive oil is quite legendary since it has been used over the centuries for multiple purposes, but due to its overpowering scent, this oil does not work well for massages. However, it is beneficial in some lotions for burns or scars. Olive is very beneficial for dry, damaged or split hair and is soothing for inflamed skin such as eczema. It has been proven to be very beneficial for rheumatic conditions and protects the body against harmful free-radical cell damage. Traditionally, olive oil has been used for stomach disorders, stimulates bile production, promotes pancreatic secretions and may even protect against stomach ulcers. The antihypertensive effects of olive oil are so powerful many users eliminated their need for blood pressure-lowering medications in just six months, according to a recent study. The "virgin" indicates it comes from the first pressing of the fruit. The "extra" means it comes from a single source. Extra virgin olive oil is particularly good for high blood pressure because it contains more vitamin E than virgin, pure or extra light varieties. Historically, olive oil has been the base for anointing oils. Olive oil is commonly used in body lotions, soaps, and hair products.

Dilution: Can be used at 100% or 25-50% dilution with another carrier oil blend.

Palm Oil comes from the fruit of the palm tree that is rich in palmitic acid, Vitamin E, Vitamin K, and magnesium. Palm oil contains saturated and unsaturated fats, vitamin E, and beta-carotene. It has antioxidant effects and is used by many to lower blood pressure. Red palm oil has recently been studied for its beneficial role in fighting heart disease and high cholesterol. Dr. Oz's website states, "...studies show that adding palm oil into the diet can remove plaque build-up in arteries and, therefore, reverse the process of plaque and prevent blockages. In fact, studies funded by the National Institutes of Health (NIH) have shown that a natural form of vitamin E called alpha-tocotrienol, which is the type found in high amounts in red palm fruit oil, can help reduce the effects of stroke by 50% by protecting your brain's nerve cells." In addition, red palm oil can improve cholesterol values and helps to maintain proper blood pressure. It is semi-solid at room temperature and must be warmed to become liquid. It is a natural source of antioxidants and is great for soap making.

Dilution: Can be used at 100% or 10% dilution with another carrier oil or carrier oil blend.

Pomegranate Seed Oil is highly sought after for beauty and skin care products. Rich in phytosterols, it is considered a treasure trove of beneficial properties for the skin because of its antioxidants, punicic acids and gallic acids. Punicic acid is an oil known as "Super CLA" or linoleic acid that is found to support healthy fat metabolism and weight loss. The oil is an excellent base for all types of skin conditions, including eczema, sunburn, dry and cracked skin and mature skin. Pomegranate Seed oil also revives the skin's elastic nature. Research has shown the oil actually to stimulate keratinocyte production, strengthening the dermis. Punicalagin, a compound found only in pomegranates, is shown to benefit the heart and blood vessels and is the major component responsible for pomegranate's antioxidant and health benefits. It not only lowers cholesterol but also lowers blood pressure and increases the speed at which heart blockages (atherosclerosis) melt away, according to research. In other studies, potent antioxidant compounds found in pomegranates have shown to reduce platelet aggregation and naturally lower blood pressure, preventing both heart attacks and strokes. The oil is rich in phytoestrogens as well, which helps women manage menopause symptoms.

Pomegranate Seed oil can be used alone or combined with a lotion or base oil such as Jojoba, Almond or Olive and then applied to the skin.

Dilution: Can be used at 100% or blended with another carrier oil at 25-50% dilution.

Pumpkin Seed Oil is a mildly rich yellow oil, containing protein, oleic acid, linoleic acid, palmitic acid, Stearic acid, Omega-3 and Omega-6 fatty acids, which are known to support brain function, and give you overall health and vitality. Pumpkin Seed oil also contains high levels of Vitamin E, as well as Vitamins A and C, Zinc, and other trace minerals and vitamins. This oil strengthens the lungs and mucous membranes and can be used as an alternative to fish oils. It is useful as a diuretic for urinary complaints, as a demulcent and as an anthelmintic to expel intestinal worms. It is readily absorbed by the skin and can be used by all skin types. Pumpkin Seed oil is fabulous for combating fine lines and makes a great moisturizer for face creams, lotions, bath oils, massage oils and other skincare products.

Dilution: Use at a 10% dilution with another carrier oil or carrier oil blend.

Rosehip Oil is called the queen of carrier oils because of its luxurious treatment for wrinkles, scars and inflamed skin. It is an excellent oil for cosmetic uses as it helps with cell regeneration by preventing premature aging and smoothing lines. In addition, Rosehip is good for eczema, psoriasis, PMS, menopause and high blood pressure. According to a study conducted and published in the European Journal of Clinical Nutrition, supplements with Rosehip significantly reduced blood pressure and LDL cholesterol. Cold-pressed from the seeds of Rosehips, its pale yellow light texture makes it a wonderful carrier oil for skin care.

Dilution: Use sparingly alone, or use at 10% dilution when blended with other carrier oils.

Safflower Oil has a slightly nutty aroma and is rich in an Omega-6 group of essential fatty acids, oleic acid, palmitic acid, linoleic acid and linolenic acid as well as Vitamin E. It has the highest percentage of unsaturated fats of all vegetable oils. Because of its light texture, Safflower oil is suitable for body massage. It has diuretic properties and is helpful for painful, inflamed joints, bruises, and sprains. This oil is also great for skin allergies and is beneficial for people who suffer from arteriosclerosis and is a good choice for those who want to improve the health of their cardiovascular system. This oil oxidizes quickly. Safflower can be used in massage blends.

Dilution: Can be used at 100% or diluted with another carrier oil blend.

Sesame Oil has a rich golden color with a bold, nutty flavor. It is a warm oil that is used for conditions such as eczema, psoriasis, and arthritis. Sesame oil is active with Vitamin A and E, minerals and lecithin. Research has shown Sesame oil enriches the blood, stimulates the blood platelet count, and is effective against spleen disorders. One website reported, "It is almost as effective as a drug for bringing down high blood pressure, and the oils also improve cholesterol levels." It is high in calcium and makes an ideal laxative for those who suffer from digestive disorders. It works great as an all-over body moisturizer or massage oil. Because of its relatively stable shelf life, it is great in body care products and facial blends. However, it needs to be mixed with another carrier oil that inhibits oxidation or an essential oil such as Benzoin. Sesame spreads easily all over the skin and leaves no greasy feeling.

Dilution: Use at 10% dilution with another carrier oil or carrier oil blend.

Shea Butter is a thick, lustrous butter (not a carrier oil) with magnificent therapeutic properties. It leaves the skin feeling smooth and healthy and combats many skin conditions including dermatitis, eczema, burns, dry skin and more. Shea butter has a very creamy consistency so you may want to warm and blend with other carrier oils for a thinner or liquid consistency if desired.

Dilution: Can be used at 100% or diluted at 25-25% with another carrier oil for blending purposes.

Sunflower Oil has high amounts of Vitamins A, D, and E as well as beneficial amounts of lecithin and unsaturated fatty acids. Its deeply nourishing benefits for the skin make it a favorite for recipes designed to treat dry, mature and damaged skin. It can be used for facial treatments and body massage as it offers satisfying softening and moisturizing properties. It also relieves the burn of sunburn. Sunflower oil is suitable for all skin types and frequently used for beauty and skin care products. It is considered an effective diuretic, helps with respiratory tract infections, especially if blended with sympathetic essential oils. This oil contains the highest level of vitamin E when compared to all the other vegetable oils. Vitamin E plays a role in normalizing blood pressure. Stores well under any condition but extreme heat and light will lessen the shelf life. It is not easily absorbed by the skin when applied and should be diluted with another carrier oil as a blend.

Dilution: Use at a 50% dilution with another carrier oil or carrier oil blend.

Walnut Oil makes an excellent emollient with moisturizing properties for dry, aged, and irritated skin. This pale yellow oil works as a balancing agent for the nervous system. A study published in the Journal of the American College of Nutrition examined walnuts and walnut oils, which contain polyunsaturated fats and their influence on blood pressure at rest and under stress and found it helps the body cope with stress by lowering resting blood pressure and blood pressure responses to stress. Previous studies showed that Omega-3 fatty acids—like the alpha linolenic acid found in walnuts and flax seeds—can reduce low-density lipoproteins (LDL) and may reduce c-reactive protein and other markers of inflammation. Walnut oil can be used for massage and aromatherapy. However, it should be diluted with another carrier oil.

Dilution: Use at 10-25% dilution with another carrier oil or carrier oil blend.

Wheat Germ Oil is high in Vitamin E, B1, B2, B3, B6, zinc, potassium, sulfur, phosphorus and other fatty acids that contain a natural antioxidant to help prevent rancidity. It can be added to other carrier oils to help to avoid rancidity and lengthen their shelf life. Wheat Germ helps with its highly nourishing oil to promote the formation of new cells, improve circulation and repair sun damaged skin. It is also used to relieve the symptoms of dermatitis, psoriasis, and eczema. Its consistency is extremely heavy and sticky which makes it not suitable to use as a carrier alone, but can be added to another carrier oil blend when mixing a massage oil. It is useful for healing scar tissue, burns, wrinkles and stretch marks. Wheat Germ is known to strengthen the nervous system internally and helps remove the fatty plaque from arteries. It strengthens dry and split hair when massaged into the split ends for several minutes before washing.

Dilution: Use with other carrier oils at 5-10% dilution. Warning: May cause sensitization in some individuals.

DO NOT USE THESE

Mineral oil and petroleum jelly should never be used as a carrier oil in therapeutic blending. These are derivatives of petroleum production from gasoline and are not of natural botanical origins. Many commercially-based cosmetics and moisturizers contain mineral oil such as baby oil because it is so inexpensive to manufacture. However, it clogs pores and prevents the skin from breathing naturally. In addition, it prevents toxins from escaping the body through perspiration and is believed to also prevent the body from properly absorbing vitamins and utilizing them, including essential oil absorption.

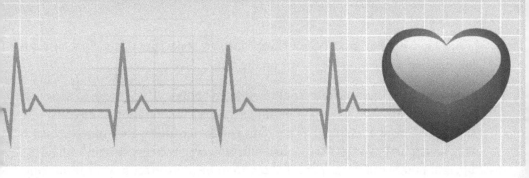

DILUTION RATE FOR YOUR CHOLESTEROL BLENDS

When creating an essential oil blend for high cholesterol, you will need to take into consideration the percentage of dilution with a carrier oil. Be careful to dilute properly to make sure your blend is safe to use and doesn't waste your precious essential oil.

The following dilution rate chart shows you the percentage of pure therapeutic essential oil to use with the number of drops of carrier oil (vegetable oil) and will help you convert essential and carrier oil measurements. Use a measuring cup or spoon for carrier oils and pipettes for measuring your essential oils.

It is important to dilute your essential oil blend with a suitable carrier oil so that you can use it on the skin over a part of the body. There are several different carrier oils as mentioned earlier, such as Sweet Almond, cold-pressed Extra Virgin Olive, Flaxseed, Avocado, Grapeseed Extract, Jojoba, etc. You will want to select the best one for your condition and skin type. Carrier oils can be purchased at a natural health food store or grocery, but check labels to make sure the one you select is cold-pressed and is suitable for use on the skin.

In general, most essential oils should be diluted between 1%-5% with a carrier oil. For topical formulas, you will typically use 1-3% concentration of essential oils. This is 6-24 drops of essential oil per ounce of carrier. Therapeutic massage blends will contain between 1%-5% essential oils. However, each essential oil will have a different number of drops per milliliter, so to be more exact in your measuring, you will want to take this into consideration, too.

For instance, if you use two to three drops of pure essential oil, you will dilute by adding about a teaspoon of carrier oil. This should be cut in half for children and senior citizens.

SIMPLE EVERYDAY DILUTION CHART

2-3 drops of Essential Oil per teaspoon of Carrier Oil
7-8 drops of Essential Oil per Tablespoon of Carrier Oil
15 drops of Essential Oil per ounce (30ml) of Carrier Oil
1 drop of essential oil = 1 tsp. of carrier oil for 1% dilution
2 drops of essential oil = 1 tsp. of carrier oil for 2% dilution
3 drops of essential oil = 1 tsp. of carrier oil for 3% dilution
4 drops of essential oil = 1 tsp. of carrier oil for 4% dilution
5 drops of essential oil = 1 tsp. of carrier oil for 5% dilution

Essential Oil	To	Carrier Oil
1 drop		¼ teaspoon
2-5 drops		1 teaspoon
4-10 drops		2 teaspoons
6-15 drops		1 Tablespoon
8-20 drops		4 teaspoons
12-30 drops		2 Tablespoons

For general purposes, a blend is applied 6 times a day for acute conditions and 3-6 times a day for chronic complaints, or as needed.

MASSAGE OIL

When you use essential oils for a massage, you will definitely need to dilute with a carrier oil. Generally, two drops of therapeutic grade essential oil should be used per teaspoon of carrier oil (follow individual recipes when available). A full body massage takes about one to two ounces of carrier oil. Any natural carrier oil (except mineral oil) is fine to use when preparing a massage blend. As a general rule, add 10-12 drops of essential oil to 30ml of carrier oil. For children and elderly, use only 5-6 drops of essential oil to 30ml of carrier oil.

QUICK CONVERSIONS FOR DILUTION

Teaspoons to Drops
1/8 teaspoon = 12.5 drops = 1/48 ounce = 5/8 ml
1/4 teaspoon = 25 drops = 1/24 ounce = 1 1/4 ml
3/4 teaspoon = 75 drops = 1/8 ounce = 3.7 ml
1 teaspoon = 100 drops = 1/6 ounce = 5 ml

ML Conversion to Ounces (approximate drops)
1 ml = 20-24 drops
3 ml = .10 ounce (approximately 60-72 drops)
6 ml = .20 ounce (approximately 120-144 drops)
9 ml = .30 ounce (approximately 180-216 drops)
12 ml = .40 ounce (approximately 240-288 drops)
24 ml = .80 ounce (approximately 480-576 drops)

Quick Conversions
3 teaspoons (tsp.) = 1 Tablespoon (Tbsp.)
2 Tablespoons (Tbsp.) = 1 ounce (oz.)
6 teaspoons (tsp.) = 1 ounce (oz.)
10 milliliter (ml) = 1/3 ounce (oz.)
15 milliliter (ml) = 1/2 ounce (oz.)
30 milliliter (ml) = 1 ounce (oz.)
10 milliliter (ml) = approximately 300 drops

1% Dilution Rate (approximate)

1 ounce carrier oil (2 Tablespoons) + 6 drops essential oil

2 ounces carrier oil (1/4 cup) + 12 drops essential oil

3 ounces carrier oil (1/3 cup) + 18 drops essential oil

4 ounces carrier oil (1/2 cup) + 24 drops (or 1 ml) essential oil

8 ounces carrier oil (1 cup) + 48 drops (or 2 ml) essential oil

2% Dilution Rate (approximate)

1 ounce carrier oil (2 Tablespoons) + 12 drops essential oil

2 ounces carrier oil (1/4 cup) + 24 drops (or 1 ml) essential oil

3 ounces carrier oil (1/3 cup) + 36 drops (or 1½ ml) essential oil

4 ounces carrier oil (1/2 cup) + 48 drops (or 2 ml) essential oil

8 ounces carrier oil (1 cup) + 96 drops (or 4 ml) essential oil

3% Dilution Rate (approximate)

1 ounce carrier oil (2 Tablespoons) + 18 drops essential oil

2 ounces carrier oil (1/4 cup) + 36 drops (or 1½ ml) essential oil

3 ounces carrier oil (1/3 cup) + 44 drops (or 2 ml) essential oil

4 ounces carrier oil (1/2 cup) + 72 drops (or 3 ml) essential oil

8 ounces carrier oil (1 cup) + 144 drops (or 6 ml) essential oil

5% Dilution Rate (approximate)

1 ounce carrier oil (2 Tablespoons) + 1.5 ml essential oil

2 ounces carrier oil (1/4 cup) + 3 ml essential oil

3 ounces carrier oil (1/3 cup) + 4.5 ml essential oil

4 ounces carrier oil (1/2 cup) + 6 ml essential oil

8 ounces carrier oil (1 cup) + 9 ml essential oil

10% Dilution Rate (approximate)

1 ounce carrier oil (2 Tablespoons) + 3 ml essential oil

2 ounces carrier oil (1/4 cup) + 6 ml essential oil

3 ounces carrier oil (1/3 cup) + 9 ml essential oil

4 ounces carrier oil (1/2 cup) + 12 ml essential oil

8 ounces carrier oil (1 cup) + 24 ml essential oil

EQUIPMENT USED FOR CREATING BLENDS FOR LOWERING CHOLESTEROL

Before getting started, you will want to gather the supplies you will need such as bottles, droppers, and containers. Below is a list of the necessary tools you will need to have on hand:

Glass Bottles preferably dark, in 5ml, 10ml, and 15ml sizes with orifice reducers (plastic dropper) can be used to make topical essential oil blends.

Plastic Bottles with a pump, squirt, or screw off top are suitable for liquid soaps, shower gels, shampoos, lotions, and conditioners. You can find these in 2-ounce, 4-ounce, and 8-ounce sizes.

Plastic or Glass Spray Bottles are great to have on hand when making room sprays, facial spritzers or cleaning solutions. You will find these in 1-ounce, 2-ounce, 4-ounce, 8-ounce and 16-ounce sizes.

Small Glass or Plastic Tubs are perfect for bath salts, facial creams, salves, scrubs or other bath blends. These come in a variety of shapes and sizes from 2-ounce to 8-ounce.

Pocket Diffusers are perfect as "personal inhalers" to carry in a pocket or purse with your favorite blend. They come with a cotton wick that saturates the essential oil inside the chamber. These are terrific for taking to work or school!

Plastic Transfer Pipettes come in different sizes and lengths for easy and precise drop measuring. They are ideal for filling small vials and for measure dropping small amounts of oils. Use these when you want to transfer oil from a large bottle into smaller bottles. They are for one-time use and should be thrown away to avoid cross-contamination.

Clear Mini Atomizers are perfect for trips. You can use these to make and share with friends and family (1ml or 2ml sizes work best).

You will need waterproof labels for your bottles, and you will want them in all shapes and sizes. Visit Online Labels for a wide variety of sizes at http://www.onlinelabels.com/.

Items such as bottles and pipettes are available online at SKS Bottle & Packaging and Rachel's Supply.

ESSENTIAL OIL PRECAUTIONS FOR TOPICAL APPLICATIONS

Do Not Use With High Blood Pressure: Camphor, Hyssop

Do Not Use These Oils Anytime: Bitter Almond, Boldo, Buchu, Cade, Calamus, Brown Camphor, Costus, Elecampane, Mustard, Pennyroyal, Rue, Sassafras, Thuja, and Vanilla

Oils That May Be Mucous Membrane Irritants: Allspice, Cinnamon, Clove Bud, Oregano, Savory, Spearmint, and Thyme (not linalool)

Oils Not Recommended For Use in Bath: Basil, Benzoin, Bergamot, Black Pepper, Clove Bud, Cinnamon, Eucalyptus, Lemon, Litsea cubeba (May Chang), Marjoram, Nutmeg, Orange, Oregano, Peppermint, Pine, Rosemary, Sage, Spearmint, Tarragon, and Thyme

Oils Not Recommended For Children Under 5 Years: Basil, Camphor, Cedarwood (*Cedrus atlantica*), Eucalyptus, Fennel, Hyssop, Geranium, Jasmine, Marjoram, Nutmeg, Rose, Rosemary, Sage, and Tarragon

Oils To Avoid With Diabetes: Angelica Root

Oils To Avoid With Epilepsy: Camphor, Eucalyptus, Fennel, Hyssop, Rosemary, Sage, and Wormwood

Oils To Avoid When Using Homeopathic Remedies: Black Pepper, Camphor, Eucalyptus, Peppermint, Rosemary, and Spearmint

Oils To Avoid With Kidney Disease: Juniper Berry

Oils To Avoid With Low Blood Pressure: Clary Sage, Lavender, Marjoram, and Ylang Ylang

Oils Not Recommended For Long Term Use (more than 10 days in a row): Black Pepper, Fennel, Juniper Berry, Marjoram, and Tarragon

Oils To Avoid During Pregnancy: Anise Star, Aniseed, Basil, Bay Laurel, Birch, Bitter Almond, Camphor, Citronella, Cistus, Clary Sage, Clove Bud, Cedarwood, Cinnamon, Cumin, Cypress, Eucalyptus, Fennel, Frankincense, Hyssop, Indian Ginger, Jasmine, Juniper Berry, Marjoram, Mugwort, Myrrh, Nutmeg, Oregano, Pennyroyal, Rosemary, Sage, Tansy, Tarragon, Thyme, and Wintergreen

Oils Not Recommended For Sensitive Skin (or should be diluted): Aniseed, Basil, Bay Laurel, Bergamot, Black Pepper, Cajeput, Camphor, Citronella, Clove Bud, Fennel, Geranium, Ginger, Grapefruit, Lemon, Lemongrass, Lime, Mandarin, Orange, Oregano, Rosemary, Peppermint, Petitgrain, Pine, Pimento Leaf, Savory, Spearmint, Spruce, Thyme, Oregano, and Wintergreen

Oils That May Be Photo-Toxic or Cause Sun Sensitivity: Angelica Root, Bergamot, Cumin, Grapefruit, Lemon, Lime, Mandarin, Melissa, Opoponax, Orange, and Verbena

Oils That May Be Potentially Toxic: Ajowan, Bitter Almond, Inula, Khella, Mugwort (Wormwood), Pennyroyal, and Sassafras

Oils Considered Very Toxic: Arnica, Boldo, Buchu, Calamus, Cascarilla, Chervil, Camphor (brown), Deer Tongue, Horseradish, Jaborandi, Mustard, Narcissus, and Rue

Oils To Avoid With History of Estrogen-Dependent Cancer: Aniseed, Basil, Clary Sage, Cypress, Fennel, Geranium, Myrrh, Pine (prostate cancer), Sage, Tarragon, and Vitex

Oils To Avoid Long-Term Use with Estrogen-Dependent Cancer: Roman Chamomile

Oils That May Increase Narcotic Effect of Alcohol: Clary Sage

ESSENTIAL OILS PRECAUTIONS FOR INHALATION

The following essential oils presented a slight risk of an increase of blood pressure temporary when administered through intense inhalation. This group mainly consists of oils high in carvone or limonene.

Oils To Avoid With High Blood Pressure: Grapefruit, Lemon, Caraway, Black Pepper, Fennel, Tarragon

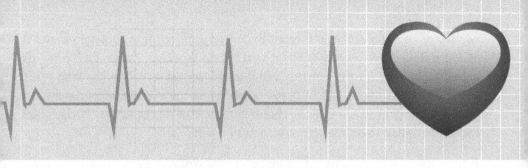

SUPPORTING RESEARCH

The following information and links are just a sampling of research being conducted on the effects of essential oils for high cholesterol. This is certainly good news for many who are seeking answers to this national health epidemic.

THE IMPACT OF LEMONGRASS OIL, AN ESSENTIAL OIL, ON SERUM CHOLESTEROL.

Elson CE, Underbakke GL, Hanson P, Sharago E, Wainberg RH, Qureshi AA.

Lemongrass essential oil tested the hypothesis that non-sterol mevalonate pathway end products lower serum cholesterol levels, we asked 22 hypercholesterolemic subjects (315 +/- 9 mg cholesterol/dl) to take a daily capsule containing 140 mg of **lemongrass oil, an essential oil rich in geraniol and citral.** The paired difference in serum cholesterol levels of subjects completing the 90-day study approached significance (P less than 0.06, 2-tailed t-test). The subjects segregated into two groups, one consisting of 14 subjects resistant to the protocol and the other comprised of 8 subjects who responded. Paired differences in cholesterol level at 30, 60 and 90 d for resistant subjects were +2 +/- 6, +2 +/- 7 and -1 +/- 6 mg/dl; paired differences for the responding subjects were -25 +/- 10 (p less than 0.05), -33 +/- 8 (p less than 0.01) and -38 +/- 10 (p less than 0.025), respectively. The paired difference (+8 +/- 4) in the cholesterol levels of six responders 90 days after the discontinuation of lemongrass oil was not significant.

Source: http://www.ncbi.nlm.nih.gov/pubmed/2586227

THE CHOLESTEROL-LOWERING PROPERTY OF CORIANDER SEEDS (CORIANDRUM SATIVUM): MECHANISM OF ACTION.

Dhanapakiam P, Joseph JM, Ramaswamy VK, Moorthi M, Kumar AS.

Coriandrum sativum (Coriander) essential oil has been documented as a traditional treatment for cholesterol and diabetes patients. In the present study, coriander seeds incorporated into diet and the effect of the administration of coriander seeds on the metabolism of lipids was studied in rats, fed with a high-fat diet and added cholesterol. The seeds had a significant hypolipidemic action. In the experimental group of rats (tissue) the level of total cholesterol and triglycerides increased significantly. There was a significant increase in beta-hydroxy, beta-methyl glutaryl-CoA reductase and plasma lecithin-cholesterol acyltransferase activity was noted in the experimental group. The level of low-density lipoprotein (LDL) + very low-density lipoprotein (VLDL) cholesterol decreased while that of high-density lipoprotein (HDL) cholesterol increased in the experimental group compared to the control group. The increased activity of plasma LCAT enhanced degradation of cholesterol to fecal bile acids, and neutral sterols appeared to account for its hypocholesterolemic effect.

Pharmacogn Mag. 2010 Jul;6(23):147-53. doi: 10.4103/0973-1296.66926.

PROTECTIVE EFFECTS OF BIOACTIVE PHYTOCHEMICALS FROM MENTHA PIPERITA WITH MULTIPLE HEALTH POTENTIALS.

Sharafi SM, Rasooli I, Owlia P, Taghizadeh M, Astaneh SD.

Mentha piperita (Peppermint) essential oil was bactericidal in order of E. coli> S. aureus > Pseudomonas aeruginosa > S. faecalis > Klebsiella pneumoniae. The oil with total phenolics of 89.43 ± 0.58 µg GAE/mg had 63.82 ± 0.05% DPPH inhibition activity with an IC (50) = 3.9 µg/ml. Lipid peroxidation inhibition was comparable to BHT and BHA. A 127% hike was noted in serum ferric-reducing antioxidant power. There was 38.3% decrease in WBC count, while platelet count showed increased levels of 214.12%. **A significant decrease in the uric acid level and cholesterol/HDL and LDL/HDL ratios were recorded.** The volatile oil displayed high cytotoxic action toward the human tumor cell line. The results of this study deserve attention with regard to antioxidative and possible anti-neoplastic chemotherapy that form a basis for future research. The essential oil of mint may be exploited as a natural source of bioactive phytochemicals bearing antimicrobial and antioxidant potentials that could be supplemented for both nutritional purposes and preservation of foods.

Source: http://www.ncbi.nlm.nih.gov/pubmed/20931070

CHOLESTEROL REDUCTION AND LACK OF GENOTOXIC OR TOXIC EFFECTS IN MICE AFTER REPEATED 21-DAY ORAL INTAKE OF LEMONGRASS (CYMBOPOGON CITRATUS) ESSENTIAL OIL.

Costa CA, Bidinotto LT, Takahira RK, Salvadori DM, Barbisan LF, Costa M.

Cymbopogon citratus (Lemongrass) Essential oil is currently used in traditional folk medicine. Although this species presents widespread use, there is no scientific data on its efficacy or safety after repeated treatments. Therefore, this work investigated the toxicity and genotoxicity of this lemongrass's essential oil (EO) in male Swiss mice. The single LD(50) based on a 24h acute oral toxicity study was found to be around 3500 mg/kg. In a repeated dose 21-day oral toxicity study, mice were randomly assigned to two control groups, saline- or Tween 80 0.01%-treated groups, or one of the three experimental groups receiving lemongrass EO (1, 10 or 100mg/kg). No significant changes in gross pathology, body weight, absolute or relative organ weights, histology (brain, heart, kidneys, liver, lungs, stomach, spleen and urinary bladder), urinalysis or clinical biochemistry were observed in EO-treated mice relative to the control groups. **Additionally, blood cholesterol was reduced after EO-treatment at the highest dose tested.** Similarly, data from the comet assay in peripheral blood cells showed no genotoxic effect from the EO. **In conclusion, our findings verified the safety of lemongrass intake at the doses used in folk medicine and indicated the beneficial effect of reducing the blood cholesterol level.** Copyright © 2011 Elsevier Ltd. All rights reserved.

HYPOLIPIDEMIC EFFECTS OF DIFFERENT ANGIOCARP PARTS OF ALPINIA ZERUMBET.

Chuang CM, Wang HE, Peng CC, Chen KC, Peng RY.

Zingiber officinale (Ginger) essential oil, in the utilization of Alpinia zerumbet (Pers.) Burtt and Smith (Zingiberaceae) (AZ), usually the angiocarps are discarded without further use. We speculate whether the angiocarps could show hypolipidemic effect.

Several diets were prepared: Alpinia seed powder (ASP); Alpinia seed powder/husk (ASH): 40/60; and Alpinia seed essential oil (ASO): 0.01-0.10%. Sprague-Dawley rats divided into 11 groups were fed these diets for eight weeks and tested for the hypolipidemic bioactivity.

The fecal neutral cholesterol excretion was increased, and the total serum triglyceride (TG) was significantly reduced from 153.7 mg/dL in the high-fat group (H) to 114.3-119.8 mg/dL by ASO; to 116.3-147.9 mg/dL by ASP, and to 116.2-145.3 mg/dL by ASH. The activity of superoxide dismutase (SOD) and glutathione peroxidase (GPX) were almost unaffected. ASO mostly raised the high-density lipoprotein (HDL) levels to 180.3-200.8 mg/dL. The low-density lipoprotein (LDL) levels were mostly reduced to 66.8-82.6 mg/dL by ASH. The level of arachidonic acid was mostly raised to 0.50-0.60% by ASO, compared with 0.37% of group H. **More importantly, the significant reduction in hepatic TG and total cholesterol (TC) implicated a crucial liver protective effect.**

ASP and ASH consisted of high crude fiber content, while ASO consisted of seed essential oil. Both the seed essential oil and the whole powder of AZ previously had been reported to possess potent hypolipidemic bioactivity. **Conclusively, the hypolipidemic effect can be attributed to the combined effect of Ginger essential oil and the crude fiber.**

SAGE LEAF EXTRACT MAY BE SAFE AND EFFECTIVE IN TREATING HYPERLIPIDEMIA

Kianbakht S, Abasi B, Perham M, Hashem Dabaghian F. Antihyperlipidemic effects of Salvia officinalis L. leaf extract in patients with hyperlipidemia: a randomized, double-blind placebo-controlled clinical trial. Phytother Res. Apr 2011; [Epub ahead of print]. doi: 10.1002/ptr.3506.

Hyperlipidemia (abnormally elevated blood lipids or lipoprotein—total and low-density lipoprotein [LDL] cholesterol, very low-density lipoprotein [VLDL], triglycerides, and chylomicrons) can cause cardiovascular disease. Primary hyperlipidemia is caused by genetic mutations and is divided into three categories: hypercholesterolemia, hypertriglyceridemia, and combined hyperlipidemia (elevated total cholesterol and triglycerides, and decreased high-density lipoprotein [HDL] cholesterol). Alternative treatments are required because some patients are resistant to current treatments. **Sage (Salvia officinalis) has antihyperlipidemic effects in vitro.** There is only one pilot clinical study that evaluates lipid levels other than blood triglyceride and VLDL. Hence, the purpose of this randomized, double-blind, placebo-controlled study was to evaluate the efficacy and safety of sage leaf extract in treating primary hyperlipidemia.

Male and female outpatients (n = 67; mean age: 56 years; mean body mass index: 29 kg/m2) with newly diagnosed primary hyperlipidemia (fasting serum triglyceride and total cholesterol levels = 240-300 mg/dL) participated in this study conducted in Iran. Patients were excluded from the study if they were taking other antihyperlipidemic agents, estrogen, steroids, beta-blockers, or thiazide. Patients were also excluded if they had cardiac disease, renal disease, hepatic disease, hematological disease, hypothyroidism, diabetes mellitus, tachycardia, vertigo, seizure, or a history of gallstones or gallbladder surgery. Sage was collected in August from the western Mazandaran province, Iran, and its identity was authenticated. The leaves were washed and then shade dried at room temperature. The dried leaves were ground into powder. The dried sage leaf powder (20 kg) was extracted with ethanol/water (80/20 v/v). The extract contained 2.16% quercetin. Patients took a dose of one 500 mg sage leaf extract capsule or a placebo capsule orally every 8 hours for two months. At baseline and study end, blood was collected, and levels of total cholesterol, triglycerides, VLDL, LDL cholesterol, HDL cholesterol, creatinine, and liver enzymes (serum glutamic-oxaloacetic transaminase [SGOT] and serum glutamic-pyruvic transaminase [SGPT]) were measured.

No drop outs and no adverse events were reported. At baseline, the levels of total cholesterol, LDL, VLDL, HDL, SGOT, SGPT, and creatinine were not significantly different between the groups. The baseline triglyceride level was significantly higher in the sage group. **At study end, sage treatment reduced total cholesterol by 19.6%, triglycerides by 22.8%, LDL by 19.7%, and VLDL by 13.3% compared with baseline. Sage increased HDL levels by 20.2% compared with baseline.** This effect was significantly different from placebo: P < 0.001 for total cholesterol, triglycerides, VLDL, and HDL, and P = 0.004 for LDL. There was no significant effect on SGOT, SGPT, and creatinine levels.

The authors conclude that since sage had no significant effects on SGOT, SGPT, and creatinine, it would not produce liver or kidney toxicity. Sage leaves had favorable effects on a variety of lipids. Thus, sage leaves may be useful for treating hypercholesterolemia and hypertriglyceridemia. Despite the positive findings, various questions remain. The mechanism of action, bioactive component, and optimal dose are unknown. Also, the study did not evaluate the duration, and specifically not the sustainability, of the beneficial effect. Results may vary for other ethnic populations with a different lifestyle and diet. Additional research is necessary to answer these questions. —Heather S. Oliff, PhD

Source: https://www.youngliving.com/export/sites/youngliving/en_US/pdfs/YL_HerbClips_Sage_06302011_1.pdf

----

THE EFFECT OF HYDRO ALCOHOLIC EXTRACT AND ESSENTIAL OIL OF HERACLEUM PERSICUM ON LIPID PROFILE IN CHOLESTEROL-FED RABBITS.

Hajhashemi V, Dashti G, Saberi S, Malekjamshidi P.

This study was designed to investigate the effect of hydroalcoholic extract and **essential oil of Heracleum persicum (Apiaceae)** on the lipid profile of male hyperlipidemic rabbits.

Thirty rabbits were randomly divided into six groups of five each. One group received standard diet and the other groups fed with a high cholesterol (2% W/W) diet for seven weeks. The vehicle, hydroalcoholic extract (500 and 1000 mg/kg), essential oil (200 l/kg), and lovastatin (5 mg/kg) were administered orally to animals, and their effects on lipid profile were evaluated.

Essential oil of H. perscum significantly (p<0.05) lowered serum triglyceride level and increased HDL-cholesterol concentration. Moreover, hydroalcoholic extract (1000 mg/kg), essential oil (200 l/kg), and lovastatin significantly (p<0.01) reduced serum concentration of total cholesterol and LDL-cholesterol.

These findings suggest that essential oil of the plant fruits may have some benefits in reducing cardiovascular risk factors.

Source: http://www.ncbi.nlm.nih.gov/pubmed/25050312

PREVENTIVE AND AMELIORATING EFFECTS OF CITRUS D-LIMONENE ON DYSLIPIDEMIA AND HYPERGLYCEMIA IN MICE WITH HIGH-FAT-DIET-INDUCED OBESITY.

Jing L, Zhang Y, Fan S, Gu M, Guan Y, Lu X, Huang C. Zhou Z.

D-limonene is a major constituent of citrus essential oil such as Grapefruit, Orange, Tangerine, Lime and Lemon, which is used in various foods as a flavoring agent. Recently, d-limonene has been reported to alleviate fatty liver induced by a high-fat diet. Here we determined the preventive and therapeutic effects of d-limonene on metabolic disorders in mice with high-fat-diet-induced obesity. In the preventive treatment, d-limonene decreased the size of white and brown adipocytes, lowered serum triglyceride (TG) and fasting blood glucose levels, and prevented liver lipid accumulations in high-fat-diet-fed C57BL/6 mice. **In the therapeutic treatment, d-limonene reduced serum TG, low-density lipoprotein cholesterol (LDL-c) and fasting blood glucose levels and glucose tolerance, and increased serum high-density lipoprotein** cholesterol (HDL-c) in obese mice. Using a reporter assay and gene expression analysis, we found that d-limonene activated peroxisome proliferator-activated receptor (PPAR)-α signaling, and inhibited liver X receptor (LXR)-β signaling. **Our data suggest that the intake of d-limonene may benefit patients with dyslipidemia and hyperglycemia and is a potential dietary supplement for preventing and ameliorating metabolic disorders.** © 2013 Elsevier B.V. All rights reserved.

Source: http://www.ncbi.nlm.nih.gov/pubmed/23838456

BAY LEAVES IMPROVE GLUCOSE AND LIPID PROFILE OF PEOPLE WITH TYPE 2 DIABETES

Alam Khan, Goher Zaman and Richard A. Anderson

Bay leaves (*Laurus nobilis*) essential oil have been shown to improve insulin function *in vitro*, but the effects on people have not been determined. The objective of this study was to determine if bay leaves may be important in the prevention and/or alleviation of type 2 diabetes. Forty people with type 2 diabetes were divided into four groups and given capsules containing 1, 2 or 3 g of ground bay leaves per day for 30 days or a placebo followed by a ten day washout period. All three levels of bay leaves reduced serum glucose with significant decreases ranging from 21 to 26% after 30 d. **Total cholesterol decreased, 20 to 24%, after 30 days with larger decreases in low-density lipoprotein (LDL) cholesterol of 32 to 40%. High-density lipoprotein (HDL) cholesterol increased 29 and 20% in the groups receiving 1 and 2 g of bay leaves, respectively. Triglycerides also decreased 34 and 25% in groups consuming 1 and 2 g of bay leaves, respectively, after 30 d.** There were no significant changes in the placebo group. In summary, this study demonstrates that consumption of bay leaves, 1 to 3 g/d for 30 days, decreases risk factors for diabetes and cardiovascular diseases and suggests that bay leaves may be beneficial for people with type 2 diabetes.

Source: http://www.ncbi.nlm.nih.gov/pmc/articles/PMC2613499/

LEMON BALM EXTRACT CAUSES POTENT ANTIHYPERGLYCEMIC AND ANTIHYPERLIPIDEMIC EFFECTS IN INSULIN-RESISTANT OBESE MICE.

Weidner C, Wowro SJ, Freiwald A, Kodelia V, Abdel-Aziz H, Kelber O, Sauer S.

Over the last decades, polyetiological metabolic diseases such as obesity and type 2 diabetes have emerged as a global epidemic. Efficient strategies for prevention and treatment include dietary intervention and the development of validated nutraceuticals. Safe extracts of edible plants provide a resource of structurally diverse molecules that can effectively interfere with multifactorial diseases. In this study, we describe the application of ethanolic lemon balm (Melissa officinalis) leaves extract for the treatment of insulin resistance and dyslipidemia in mice. We show that lemon balm extract (LBE) activates the peroxisome proliferator-activated receptors (PPARs), which have key roles in the regulation of whole-body glucose and lipid metabolism. Application of LBE (0.6 mg/mL) to human primary adipocytes resulted in specific peroxisome proliferator-activated receptor target gene expression. LBE treatment of insulin-resistant high-fat-diet-fed C57BL/6 mice (200 mg/kg/day) for six weeks considerably reduced hyperglycemia and insulin resistance, plasma triacylglycerol, non-esterified fatty acids and LDL/VLDL cholesterol levels. Taken together, ethanolic lemon balm extract can potentially be used to prevent or concomitantly treat type 2 diabetes and associated disorders such as dyslipidemia and hypercholesterolemia. © 2013 WILEY-VCH Verlag GmbH & Co. KGaA, Weinheim.

Source: http://www.ncbi.nlm.nih.gov/pubmed/24272914

DEHYDRATION DURING FASTING INCREASES SERUM LIPIDS AND LIPOPROTEINS.

Campbell NR, Wickert W, Magner P. Shumak SL

The study was an open, prospective, randomized cross-over design to determine if dehydration during fasting increases lipid concentrations. Fifteen healthy subjects participated, 1 of whom did not complete the study. The subjects fasted once with no fluid replacement and once with salt and water supplementation. Following both fasts, blood was drawn for lipid assessments. **Compared to fasting with fluid and salt replacement, fasting with no fluids was associated with higher (mean, 95% confidence interval) total serum cholesterol (8.1%, 4.3-11.9%), HDL cholesterol (7.5%, 1.8-13.1%), LDL cholesterol (10.5%, 2.2-18.8%), apolipoprotein A-1 (8.9%, 5.0-12.8%), and apolipoprotein B (10.5%, 5.2-15.8%). The change in serum triglycerides was not statistically significant (12.4%,-0.5-25.3%).** There was a greater reduction in body weight during fasting with fluid restriction compared to fasting with salt and water supplementation (1.8%, 1.3-2.2%). Fasting with fluid restriction results in significantly higher lipid levels and, therefore, variation in hydration of patients could contribute to fluctuation in lipid levels of patients. Care should be taken to ensure that patients are in a standard state of hydration during the assessment of lipid levels. We recommend: 1) that patients fast no longer than 12 h, and 2) that, during fasting, patients avoid unnecessary physical activity, avoid hot, dry environments, ensure a liberal intake of water, and avoid diuretic substances such as caffeine.

EFFECTS OF CASSIA TORA FIBER SUPPLEMENT ON SERUM LIPIDS IN KOREAN DIABETIC PATIENTS.

Cho SH, Kim TH, Lee NH, Son HS, Cho IJ, Ha TY.

Cassia tora fiber supplement consisting of 2 g of soluble fiber extracted from Cassia semen (C. tora L.), 200 mg of alpha-tocopherol, 500 mg of ascorbic acid, and 300 mg of maltodextrin was formulated in a pack, and given to 15 type II diabetic subjects (seven men and eight women 57.1 +/- 2.9 years old) with instructions to take two packs per day for 2 months. Placebo contained maltodextrin only with a little brown caramel color. Lifestyle factors and dietary intakes of the subjects were not altered during the 2-month period. Serum total cholesterol was moderately (P < .1) decreased in the C. tora group compared with the age- and gender-matched placebo group, as was the ratio of apolipoprotein B to apolipoprotein A1 (P < .1). Levels of serum triglycerides and low-density lipoprotein-cholesterol tended to decrease more in the C. tora-supplemented group than in the placebo group. Serum alpha-tocopherol was increased (P < .01) but lipid peroxides were not significantly lower in the C. tora group. Fasting blood glucose, hemoglobin A1c, blood urea nitrogen, creatinine, and activities of serum aspartate aminotransferase and alanine aminotransferase were not changed by the fiber supplement. We concluded that C. tora supplements could help improve serum lipid status in type II diabetic subjects without serious adverse effects.

Source: https://www.ncbi.nlm.nih.gov/pubmed/16176140

———

BIOACTIVITY OF ESSENTIAL OILS AND THEIR VOLATILE AROMA COMPONENTS: REVIEW

Hamdy A.E. Shaabana , Ahmed H. El-Ghoraba, and Takayuki Shibamotob

National Research Center, Flavor and Aroma Department, Dokki, Cairo, Egypt; b Department of Environmental Toxicology, University of California, Davis, CA 95616, USA (Received 31 October 2011; final form 5 December 2011)

This review discusses various biological activities of essential oils and their components that have been reported in scientific references. Antioxidant activity is one of the most intensively studied subjects in essential oil research because oxidation damages various biological substances and subsequently causes many diseases. Inhalation of the volatiles of lavender and monarda essential oils reduced the cholesterol content in the aorta and also reduced atherosclerotic plaques but had no effect on the blood cholesterol level (123).

Source: http://dx.doi.org/10.1080/10412905.2012.659528

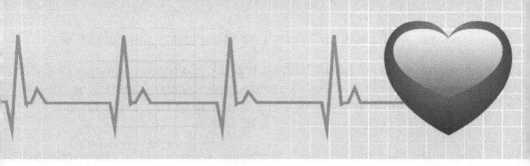

BIBLIOGRAPHY

Aourell M, Skoog M, Carleson J 2005 Effects of Swedish massage on blood pressure. Complementary Therapies in Clinical Practice 11:242-246

Aviram M, Dornfeld L, Rosenblat M, et al. Pomegranate juice consumption reduces oxidative stress, atherogenic modifications to LDL, and platelet aggregation:studies in humans and in atherosclerotic apolipoprotein E-deficient mice. Am J Clin Nutr 2000;71(5):1062-76. Aviram M, Dornfeld L. Pomegranate juice consumption inhibits serum angiotensin converting enzyme activity and reduces systolic blood pressure. Atherosclerosis 2001;158(1):195-8.

Aydin Y, Kutlay O, Ari S et al. 2007 Hypotensive effects of carvacrol on the blood pressure of normotensive rats.

Battaglia, Salvatore, 2007, The Complete Guide to Aromatherapy, The Healing Arts Press

Battaglia Salvatore, 1997, The complete guide to aromatherapy. The Perfect Potion, Virginia, Queensland

Caujolle F, Franck C 1945a Pharmacodynamic actions of clary sage and condiment sage. Comptes Rendues Société Biologique 139:1109-1110

Clarke, Sue, 2008, Essential Chemistry for Aromatherapy, Elsevier Limited

Chobanian AV, et al. and the National High Blood Pressure Education Program Coordinating Committee. The seventh report of the Joint National Committee on Prevention, Detection, Evaluation, and Treatment of High Blood Pressure: The JNC 7 report. JAMA. 2003;298:2560-2572.

Christensen BV, Lynch HJ 1937 A comparative study of the pharmacological actions of natural and synthetic camphor.

Coombs HC, Pike FH 1931 Respiratory and cardiovascular changes in the cat during convulsions of experimental origin. The American Journal of Physiology 97:92-106

Davis P 1999 Aromatherapy an A-Z. CW Daniel, Saffron Walden

Dawson AN, Walser B, Jafarzadeh M et al. 2004 Topical analgesics and blood pressure during static contraction in humans. Medicine & Science in Sports & Exercise 36:632-638

Dayawansa S, Umeno K, Takakura H et al. 2003 Autonomic responses during inhalation of natural fragrance of cedrol in humans. Autonomic Neuroscience 108:79-86

De-Oliveira AC, Ribeiro-Pinto LF, Otto SS, Goncalves A, Paumgartten FJ. Induction of liver monooxygenase by beta-myrcene. Toxicology . 1997;124(2):135-140

Fandohan P, Gnonlonfin B, Laleye A, Gbenou JD, Darboux R, Moudachirou M. Toxicity and gastric tolerance of essential oils from Cymbopogon citratus, Ocimum gratissimum and Ocimum basilicum in Wistar rats. Food Chem Toxicol . 2008;46(7):2493-2497

Franchomme P, Pénöel D 1990 L'aromathérapie exactement. Jollois, Limoges

Futami T 1984 [Actions and mechanisms of counterirritants on the muscular circulation]. Nippon Yakurigaku Zasshi 83:219-226

Gattefosse, M. (1992): Gattefosse's Aromatherapy (translated by Tisserand, R). Saffron Walden, C W Daniel.

Gaziano JM, Ridker PM, Libby P. Primary and secondary prevention of coronary heart disease. In: Bonow RO, Mann DL, Zipes DP, Libby P, eds. Braunwald's Heart Disease: A Textbook of Cardiovascular Medicine. 9th ed. Saunders; 2011:chap 49.

Goldstein LB, Bushnell CD, Adams RJ, et al. Guidelines for the primary prevention of stroke: a guideline for healthcare professionals from the American Heart Association/American Stroke Association. Stroke. 2011 Feb;42:517-84.

Greenberg B and Kahn AM. Clinical assessment of heart failure. In: Bonow RO, Mann DL, Zipes DP, Libby P, eds. Braunwald's Heart Disease: A Textbook of Cardiovascular Medicine. 9th ed. Saunders; 2011:chap 26.

Haze S, Sakai K, Gozu Y 2002 Effects of fragrance inhalation on sympathetic activity in normal adults. Japanese

Hills JM, Aaronson PI 1991 The mechanism of action of peppermint oil on gastrointestinal smooth muscle.

Jessup M, Abraham WT, Casey DE, Feldman AM, Francis GS, Ganiats TG, et al. 2009 focused update: ACCF/AHA Guidelines for the Diagnosis and Management of Heart Failure in Adults: a report of the American College of Cardiology Foundation/American Heart Association Task Force on Practice Guidelines: developed in collaboration with the International Society for Heart and Lung Transplantation. Circulation. 2009 Apr 14;119(14):1977-2016. Epub 2009 Mar 26.

Joint National Committee on Detection, Evaluation, and Treatment of Blood Pressure. The seventh report of the joint national committee on detection, evaluation, and treatment of blood pressure. NIH Publication No. 03-5233, May 2003.

Journal of the American Pharmaceutical Association 26:786-96

Journal of Pharmacology 90:247-253Heuberger E, Hongratanaworakit T, Bohm C et al. 2001 Effects of chiral fragrances on human autonomic nervous system parameters and self-evaluation. Chemical Senses 26:281-292

Kaplan NM. Systemic hypertension: Treatment. In: Bonow RO, Mann DL, Zipes DP, Libby P, eds. Braunwald's Heart Disease: A Textbook of Cardiovascular Medicine. 9th ed. Philadelphia, Pa: Saunders Elsevier; 2011:chap 46.

Kulieva ZT 1980 [Analgesic, hypotensive and cardiotonic action of the essential oil of thyme growing in Azerbaijan].

Lahlou S, Figueiredo AF, Magalhães PJ et al. 2002 Cardiovascular effects of 1,8-cineole, a terpenoid oxide present in many plant essential oils, in normotensive rats. Canadian Journal of Physiology & Pharmacology 80:1125-1131

Lahlou S, Magalhaes PJ, de Siqueira RJ et al. 2005 Cardiovascular effects of the essential oil of Aniba candelilla bark in normotensive rats. Journal of Cardiovascular Pharmacology 46:412-421

Magyar J, Szentandrassy N, Banyasz T et al. 2004 Effects of terpenoid phenol derivatives on calcium current in canine and human ventricular cardiomyocytes. European Journal of Pharmacology 487:29-36

Mant J, Al-Mohammad A, Swain S, Laramée P; Guideline Development Group. Management of chronic heart failure in adults: a synopsis of the National Institute For Health and Clinical Excellence guideline. Ann Intern Med. 2011 Aug16;155(4):252-9.

McNamara ME, Burnham DC, Smith C et al. 2003 The effects of back massage before diagnostic cardiac catheterization. Alternative Therapies in Health & Medicine 9:50-57

Mercola.com, Dr. Paul J. Rosch interview with Dr. John Laragh, Why the Treatment of Hypertension Has Become Such a Deplorable Fiasco, Part I, (Accessed 9/2/08)

Mojay, Gabriel, 1997, Aromatherapy for Healing the Spirit, Gaia Books Ltd

Northover BJ, Verghese J 1962 The pharmacology of certain terpene alcohols and oxides. Journal of Scientific & Industrial Research 21C:342-345

Peng SM, Koo M, Yu ZR., 2009 Jan, Effects of music and essential oil inhalation on cardiac autonomic balance in healthy individuals, J Altern Complement Med, 15(1):53-7

Pitman V 2004 Aromatherapy: a practical approach. Nelson Thornes, Cheltenham

Ragan BG, Nelson AJ, Foreman JH et al. 2004 Effects of a menthol-based analgesic balm on pressor responses evoked from muscle afferents in cats. American Journal of Veterinary Research 65:1204-1210

Riegel B, Moser DK, Anker SD, et al.; American Heart Association Council on Cardiovascular Nursing; American Heart Association Council on Clinical Cardiology; American Heart Association Council on Nutrition, Physical Activity, and Metabolism; American Heart Association Interdisciplinary Council on Quality of Care and Outcomes Research. State of the science: promoting self-care in persons with heart failure: a scientific statement from the American Heart Association. Circulation. 2009 Sep 22;120(12):1141-63.

Rose, J. (1994): Guide to essential oils. San Francisco, CA. Jeanne Rose Aromatherapy.

Seo JY., 2009 Jun, The effects of aromatherapy on stress and stress responses in adolescents, J Korean Acad Nursing, 39(3):357-65.

Tiran, D. (1996): Aromatherapy in midwifery practice. London, Bailliere Tindall.

Tisserand, R. (1994, 1977): The Art of Aromatherapy. Saffron Walden, The C W Daniel Co Ltd.

Tisserand, R. and Balacs, T. (1995): Essential oil safety. London, Churchill Livingstone.

Todorov S, Philianos S, Petkov V et al. 1984 Experimental pharmacological study of three species from genus Salvia.

Totilo, Rebecca Park, 2013, Therapeutic Blending With Essential Oil, Rebecca at the Well Foundation

Touvay C, Vilain B, Carre C et al. 1995 Effect of limonene and sobrerol on monocrotaline-induced lung alterations and pulmonary hypertension. International Archives of Allergy & Immunology 107:272-274Valnet J 1964 Aromathérapie. Librairie Maloine, Paris (English translation: Valnet J 1990 The practice of aromatherapy. CW Daniel, Saffron Walden)

Victor RG. Arterial hypertension. In: Goldman L, Schafer AI, eds. Cecil Medicine. 24th ed. Saunders; 2011:chap 67, 220.

Victor RG. Systemic hypertension: Mechanisms and diagnosis. In: Bonow RO, Mann DL, Zipes DP, Libby P, eds. Braunwald's Heart Disease: A Textbook of Cardiovascular Medicine. 9th ed. Philadelphia, Pa: Saunders Elsevier; 2011:chap 45.

OTHER BOOKS
BY
REBECCA PARK TOTILO

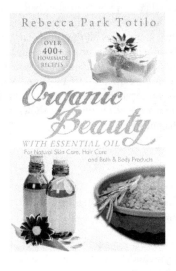

Organic Beauty With Essential Oil: Over 400+ Homemade Recipes for Natural Skin Care, Hair Care and Bath & Body Products

Sweep aside all those harmful chemically-based cosmetics and make your own organic bath and body products at home with the magic of potent essential oils! In this book, you'll find a luxurious array of over 400 Eco-friendly recipes that call for breathtaking fragrances and soothing, rich organic ingredients satisfying you head to toe. Included you'll find helpful can have the confidence knowing which essential oil to use and how much when creating your own body scrub, lip butter, or lotion bar! Discover how easy it is to make bath treats like fragrant shower gels, dreamy bubble baths, luscious creams and lotions, deep cleansing masks and facials for literally pennies using only a few essential oils and ingredients from your own kitchen with Organic Beauty with Essential Oil.

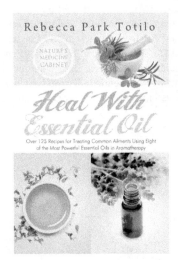

Heal With Essential Oil: Nature's Medicine Cabinet

Using essential oils drawn from nature's own medicine cabinet of flowers, trees, seeds and roots, man can tap into God's healing power to heal oneself from almost any pain. Find relief from many conditions and rejuvenate the body. With over 125 recipes, this practical guide will walk you through in the most easy-to-understand form how to treat common ailments with your essential oils for everyday living. Filled with practical advice on therapeutic blending of oils and safety, a directory of the most effective oils for common ailments and easy to follow remedies chart, and prescriptive blends for aches, pains and sicknesses.

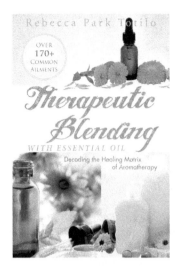

Therapeutic Blending With Essential Oil: Decoding the Healing Matrix of Aromatherapy

Therapeutic Blending With Essential Oil unlocks the healing power of essential oils and guides you through the intricate matrix of aromatherapy, with a compilation of over 170 common ailments. Discover how to properly formulate a blend for any physical or emotional symptom with easy to follow customizable recipes. Now, you can make your own personalized massage oils, hand and body lotions, bath gels, compresses, salve ointments, smelling salts, nasal inhalers and more. This exhaustive guide takes all the guesswork out of blending essential oils from how many drops to include in a blend, to working with and measuring thick oils, to how often to apply it for acute or chronic conditions. It also shows you how to create a single blend for multiple conditions. Even if you run out of oil for a favorite recipe, this book shows you how to substitute it with another oil.

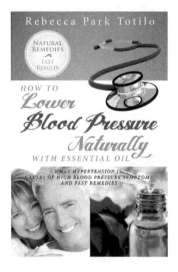

How To Lower Blood Pressure Naturally With Essential Oil: What Hypertension Is, Causes of High Pressure Symptoms and Fast Remedies

One out of three adults have it, and another one-third don't realize it. Oftentimes, it goes undetected for years. Even those who take multiple medications for it still don't have it under control. It's no secret -- high blood pressure is rampant in America. High blood pressure, or hypertension, has become a household term. Between balancing meds and monitoring diets though, are the true causes -- and best treatments -- hidden in the shadows? In How to Lower Blood Pressure Naturally With Essential Oil, Rebecca Park Totilo sheds light on what high blood pressure is, the causes and symptoms of high blood pressure, and which essential oils regulate blood pressure and how to use essential oils as a natural, alternative method.

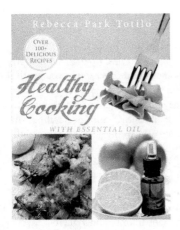

Healthy Cooking with Essential Oil

Imagine transforming an everyday dish into something extraordinary using only a drop or two of essential oil can enliven everything from soups, salads, to main dishes and desserts. Boasting flavor and fragrance, these intense essences can turn a dull, boring meal into something appetizing and delicious. Essential oils are fun, easy-to-use and beneficial, compared to the traditional stale, dried herbs and spices found in most pantries today. Healthy food should never be thought of as mere fuel for the body, it should be enjoyed as a multi-sensory experience that brings therapeutic value as well as nourishment. For years we have limited the use of essential oils to scented candles and soaps, in the belief that they were unsafe to consume (and some are!). However, more people are realizing the value of using pure essential oils to enhance their diet. In Healthy Cooking With Essential Oil, you will learn how cooking with essential oils can open up a wealth of creative opportunities in the kitchen.

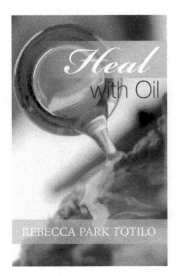

Heal With Oil: How to Use the Essential Oils of Ancient Scripture

During ancient times, spices, resins and other aromatics were an integral part of the Hebraic culture. People of the Holy Land understood the use of fragrant plants in maintaining wellness and physical healing, as well as the plant's oil to enhance their spiritual state in worship, prayer and confession, and for cleansing and purification from sin. Since the creation, fragrant oils have been inhaled, applied to the body, and taken internally in which the benefits extended to every aspect of their being. Buried within the passages of scriptures lies a hidden treasure – possibly every man's answer to illness and disease. Now you can learn their secret and discover how to transform your life and walk in divine health.

Anoint with Oil

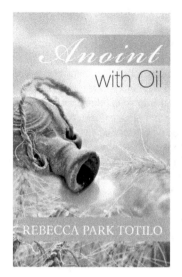

If you were taught by church leaders that anointing with oil ceased during Old Testament times, or that it is simply "symbolic" and has no power or significance today, you may be missing beauty and depth in your spiritual journey. Anointing with oil brings real benefits into your life, such as promotion, discernment, sensitivity, fruitfulness, and declaration. In Anoint With Oil, Rebecca Park Totilo shares an aromatic and sacred expedition through the scriptures, showing the purpose of anointing with oil, the methods used in the Bible and their symbolism, the ingredients of the holy anointing oil, and the uses of essential oils mentioned in the Old and New Testaments. Discover new scents within these pages and find out: – Why the right ear, right thumb, and right big toe? – What is the mysterious fifth ingredient of the holy anointing oil? – Which oils did Jesus anoint with? – Who performs the anointing ritual? – How can I benefit from anointing with oil?

CPSIA information can be obtained
at www.ICGtesting.com
Printed in the USA
BVHW081014200219
540731BV00027B/1616/P